# Better Health with AI

# Better Health with AI

## Your Roadmap to Results

**Earl J. Campazzi, Jr., M.D., M.P.H.**

with

Dominic Giovanetti, Nika Wolfs,
Lia Love, and Reagan Daly

Cover Designer
Gregory J. Del Deo

# Laura Yorke

Editor

Preliminary editing

by

**Abigail Ornellas, Ph.D., Editage**

**Dr. Vonda, FirstEditing**


Illustrations by Editage

## To Julie:

Julie is the perfect wife for me. She is brilliant and almost always by my side. She prefers to work behind the scenes but speaks her mind. Julie introduced me to AI and was among the first to recognize its potential in healthcare.

With love, respect, and awe,

Earl

**Copyright and Disclaimer**



This book contains information that is included to help the readers be better-informed consumers of healthcare. It is presented for educational and informational purposes only. This book, audiobook, and e-book are not intended to be a substitute for the medical advice of a licensed physician or medical professional, or diagnosis or treatment. They also are not intended to provide the legal advice of an attorney, or the professional advice of a financial planner. This book is based on the author's experiences, research, and viewpoints. Always consult your doctor about your individual needs about any matter relating to your health or illness.

Library of Congress Control Number: 2025918862
Hardcover ISBN: 979-8-9930227-1-0
Paperback ISBN: 979-8-9930227-0-3
e-book ISBN: 979-8-9930227-2-7
Audiobook ISBN: 979-8-9930227-3-4

Published in the United States of America
Printed in the United States of America

**Limitation of Liability/Disclaimer of Warranty:** While the publisher, author, editors, and contributors have used their best efforts in the preparation of this book, they make no representations or warranties with respect to the accuracy, reliability, suitability, or completeness of the contents of this book and specifically disclaim any implied warranties of merchantability or fitness for a particular purpose. Please note that medical research and treatment are continually evolving. No warranty may be created or extended by advertisements, marketing, sales representatives, or sales materials. The advice and strategies herein may not be suitable for your situation. You should consult with multiple medical professionals and obtain opinions regarding your health and condition, where appropriate. Considering the complexity of medicine, getting multiple opinions and consulting specialists in several areas might improve your care. The publisher, author, editors, and contributors shall not be liable for any damages or losses, including but not limited to special, incidental, consequential, direct, indirect, or other damages whatsoever arising from the use of information presented in this book. Readers should be aware that internet websites offered as citations and/or sources for further information may have changed or become unavailable. This limitation of liability shall apply to the fullest extent permitted by law.

If you're an educator seeking to utilize content from this book, please send your request for permission to mail@campazzi.com. Your request should include your name, the institution you're affiliated with, the intended purpose of use, and the scope of the material you wish to use. This process helps us ensure that the book's content is used appropriately and responsibly in educational contexts.

# TABLE OF CONTENTS

# INTRODUCTION

Living is like flying a plane with unreliable instruments. Paper cuts really hurt, yet you won't feel a small cancer. This mismatch between how we feel and our actual health doesn't always exist. Often, feeling well means we are well. But when the two don't match—when we feel fine despite growing health problems—it is unhealthy and can be dangerous.

## When Your Body's Warning System Fails

Let's use thyroid disorders as an example, given they affect about 12% of people in their lifetime, according to the American Thyroid Association. Your thyroid, a tiny gland in your neck, regulates nearly every cell, influencing your energy, mood, and metabolism. When it stops working right, the signs are hard to see because they develop slowly.

If your thyroid slows down, you might chalk up months of fatigue to stress or attribute unexpected weight gain to aging. You might think you're always cold because of poor blood flow. These symptoms emerge so gradually that you may not notice subtle changes, getting used to feeling less than your best over time. You don't know something is wrong.

Once we diagnose a thyroid issue, in most cases a single daily pill helps thyroid patients regain their energy and well-being. Within 3 weeks, it can feel like someone turned the lights back on. Many patients look back and think, "That explains why I've felt bad for months." Of course, there are times when thyroid disease treatment isn't that easy.

Now let's consider heart disease, the leading cause of death in the United States. Heart disease is harder to prevent than thyroid disease because the heart can develop many different problems, while thyroid issues are more straightforward. You may have heard about seemingly healthy people suffering sudden cardiac events in their 50s or 60s. We often think these deaths happen randomly—like being hit by lightning. But that's not true. Most sudden deaths weren't random. They came with warning signs that went unnoticed for years.

Shifts in blood pressure, heart rate, sleep patterns, and your ability to recover from exercise can signal heart issues over time. These can slowly get worse over months or years before a heart problem happens. But our body's warning system rarely tells us about these changes. Often, we don't notice until it is late or too late.

## How AI Changes Everything

Here's where artificial intelligence (AI) transforms healthcare by analyzing data from wearables like smartwatches, Oura Rings, and Fitbit trackers. It also uses data from smart scales and lab tests. AI detects patterns we often miss, like a heart rate slowing over 6–8 weeks alongside sleep disturbances, which may suggest thyroid concerns. Here are some other signs AI can notice:

- Small heart rhythm changes could signal heart disease starting
- Sleep problems might show early metabolism issues
- Poor recovery after exercise could signal many health problems

If you're worried AI sounds too complicated, don't be—it's simpler than using your smartphone. AI can help find people at risk. It can help them change lifestyle choices. It can encourage medical care. It can suggest tests to doctors. Doctors will still make final decisions. Patients will still make their own choices. But both will benefit from finding health changes earlier than our senses can catch.

## Understanding AI and How It Can Help You

To grasp how AI works, let's first explore human intelligence. We need to think about what AI is and what it isn't.

### The Human Intelligence We Can't Replicate

Human intelligence is remarkably intricate and multifaceted. I recall my grandmother's love during my childhood, when my family faced a challenging time. She knew exactly what I needed without being told: hugs, support, structure, and home cooking. Was knowing what was needed and how to provide it intelligence? Absolutely, in the most profound human sense—a sense that AI simply cannot replicate.

This distinctly human intelligence encompasses common sense, intuition, emotional understanding, empathy, and the deep connections we build with each other. AI doesn't have this heart.

### What AI Actually Is

At its core, AI focuses on analyzing data, functioning as an advanced computer system. These programs have been trained on huge amounts of data. Think of all the medical books and journals you can imagine. AI has read them all.

Think of AI as a category of different tools that all learn from massive datasets—collections of text, images, and information gathered from across the internet and specialized sources. Regular computer programs follow strict rules: if you ask the same question twice, you get the exact same answer. AI is different. It learns patterns from all that data and uses those patterns to understand your questions and generate responses that feel natural and conversational, almost like talking to a knowledgeable friend.

AI comes in many forms. You've probably heard of the large language models (LLMs) with familiar names like Grok, ChatGPT, Claude, and Gemini—these are the ones that chat with you. But AI goes far beyond conversation. There's an ever-increasing number of specialty apps for consumer health tracking and coaching. AI makes medical instruments work better, like enhancing what doctors see during colonoscopies. Software helps radiologists read mammograms and X-rays more accurately. Programs analyze raw DNA data and present it as understandable reports. As a consumer, you can use AI to understand a new diagnosis, research articles about a serious disease you or a loved one is facing, or find the best doctors and hospitals for a particular illness.

It's springtime for AI in healthcare—new tools and applications are sprouting like wildflowers in a meadow. My goal is to give you a solid overview of what's available now and show you how to use AI prompts to stay updated as this technology keeps evolving.

As I read through my book one final time before printing, something struck me: I kept repeating versions of "see your doctor" or "AI doesn't replace your doctor" throughout these pages. Four or five times, I shared stories about people who got into real trouble by relying on AI instead of getting proper medical care. I purposely left all of these warnings in, even though it might seem repetitive.

Here's why: AI is incredibly slick. It's so smooth and confident that it can convince you it's an expert—and even make you feel like an expert too. Think about whatever you do well. You're probably much better at it today than when you started, right? It likely took months or years to reach your current skill level. As a doctor, I can tell within 60 seconds of walking into an exam room whether a patient is seriously sick and needs urgent care, or whether we're dealing with something we can prevent or manage over time. I couldn't do that early in my career. Can you relate? Do you have that kind of instinct in your own work?

That's my concern with this book. I genuinely believe I'm doing something valuable by helping you understand and use AI for your health. But I also worry it's a bit like handing a 16-year-old boy the keys to a Corvette—it's powerful, exciting technology, and in the wrong hands or used the wrong way, that power could cause harm. My hope is that by understanding both AI's capabilities and its very real limitations, you'll use this tool wisely and safely, always keeping your healthcare team in the driver's seat for the serious decisions.

## AI's Special Health Powers

AI can tackle both straightforward and complex health questions, such as "Why is my heart beating irregularly, and what should I do?" But if you mentioned your age or medications earlier, it will give you a more personal and better answer. It can also study data from your fitness tracker and smart scale. It looks for small changes in your heart rate or sleep. These changes could signal health problems.

The main job of AI for your health is to see the big picture. It figures out what might be wrong with you. Or it finds out how you could be healthier. There is so much data available on your watch, phone, scale, and medical tests. It's nearly impossible for most people to spot important patterns. Even doctors struggle with this.

But finding patterns is just the start. AI can also search through tons of research. It does this better than search engines ever could. You can customize its search. It can coach you through weight loss or exercise programs.

It tailors advice to your specific needs. For example, AI will warn you when you're falling off your healthy habits. Or when you're exercising too much with the best of intentions, it can prevent overtraining by encouraging you to get more rest and sleep.

Tracking creates accountability and leads to better results. This is called the Hawthorne effect—the tendency to improve when you know you're being watched. When you monitor your health metrics, you become both the watcher and the watched. This creates a positive cycle that often leads to healthier choices.

In addition to preventing potential health risks, AI can suggest personal solutions. AI aims to be your health ally. This book tries to make it work for everyone, not just tech-savvy people.

## Important Limits to Remember

But here's what else AI isn't: It's not a doctor, and it's not perfect. Of course, doctors aren't perfect either—they have their own biases and gaps in knowledge.

Another flaw AI has is that it's based on medical studies that can be biased. Historically, clinical trials have left out many women and minorities. Fortunately, more women have been included since the 1990s thanks to new laws like the NIH Revitalization Act of 1993, but minorities are still underrepresented in many studies.

This means AI's advice might not fit everyone perfectly, but we'll teach you how to spot and fix these gaps. That means AI trained on that data might not give perfect advice for all groups. To check this, ask the AI: "How might this advice change for someone of [your background]?" And always run it by your doctor, who knows your full story.

Also, AI cannot feel your emotional stress or understand the complex personal reasons behind your symptoms. It provides facts but can't replace human judgment. This is especially true in mental health, where experts still debate AI's proper role.

When AI misses the bigger picture—like why you're tired beyond what the data shows—it's because it doesn't understand the messy, emotional parts of human life. It remains a tool that needs human guidance, especially from medical professionals.

There's another crucial limitation we need to discuss: Sometimes AI makes things up. The technical term is hallucination, but what it means is that AI can confidently give you wrong information, including fake medical studies that sound real but don't exist. This happens because AI predicts what words should come next based on patterns it learned, not because it actually knows the facts.

Here's the good news—you can catch most of these mistakes. Think of it like getting a second opinion, which you'd naturally do for important health decisions. Here are practical ways to verify what AI tells you. You don't need to use all of these methods every time—picking one or two is usually enough to feel confident about the information:

**Check with multiple AI systems.** Ask the same health question to two or three different AI programs (like ChatGPT,

Claude, or Gemini). If they all give similar answers, that's reassuring. If they disagree, that's your cue to dig deeper or ask your doctor.

**Request the evidence.** Always ask AI for references to support its health claims. Real medical studies have something called a DOI—a digital object identifier—which is like a permanent address for the research paper. When AI gives you a reference with a DOI (it looks like: https://doi.org/10.1234/ABCD), click on it. It should take you to the actual study. If the link doesn't work or goes nowhere, the reference might be fake—that happens more than occasionally with AI.

**Deal with paywalls.** Sometimes you'll click on a real study and hit a paywall asking for $30 or more to read it. Don't panic and definitely don't pay—you can usually find what you need for free. Here's how: First, try adding "PMC" (PubMed Central) to your search, since the government makes many studies available for free there. You can also search for the exact title of the paper in Google Scholar, which often shows free PDF versions. Look for "View PDF" or "Full Text" links. Remember, most medical questions have been studied multiple times, so if one paper costs money, another one on the same topic is probably free. The NIH and CDC websites also summarize research findings in plain language without charging anything.

**Verify the references.** Medical research papers can be tough to read, even for doctors. But you don't need to understand every word. Start with the abstract (the summary at the beginning) or jump to the conclusion at the end. Check if the paper actually says what the AI claimed it said. Here's a trick: Copy the abstract into a different AI and ask: "Does this study support the claim that [whatever the first AI told you]?" This gives you another perspective.

**Do your own spot-check.** Take key claims from the AI and search for them yourself. If AI says a certain supplement helps with sleep, search for "[supplement name] sleep studies" and see what comes up. Reputable health websites like Mayo Clinic, Cleveland Clinic, or NIH often have reliable information you can understand.

**One more thing:** Finally, just like you'd read reviews before trying a new restaurant, choose health apps that are backed by research from trusted places like universities or medical centers.

**The golden rule:** For any health decision—even something that seems minor like starting a new vitamin—double-check AI's advice using at least one of these methods, and always talk to your doctor or nurse practitioner before making changes. Your health is too important to rely on a single source, even a smart one.

These tools sound helpful, but cost can be a real barrier for many folks. The good news is there are free options like smartphone health apps that come preinstalled, or low-cost genetic tests starting around $100. If money's tight, check with community health centers—they often have programs for free screenings or discounted wearables. Your doctor might know about assistance programs too, so don't hesitate to ask.

Remember, AI is like a well-read assistant who sometimes confuses things they've read. It's incredibly helpful for organizing information and spotting patterns, but it needs you to verify the important stuff. This extra step takes a few minutes but could save you from following bad advice.

As we explore using AI for your health throughout this book, think of it as a smart partner without real feelings. AI is a bit like Rain Man—Dustin Hofman's character who could do amazing calculations but couldn't connect emotionally with people. When you ask AI for help with a diagnosis, it might say "I'm sorry to hear that," but can a computer program actually feel sorry? I don't think so—not yet anyway. AI is programmed to sound friendly and supportive, but underneath it's just doing very sophisticated calculations. It's excellent at tracking your health data and spotting patterns, but it can't give you the caring connection that comes from another human being. Understanding this helps you use AI's strengths without expecting things it can't deliver.

## Protecting Your Privacy While Getting Better Care

### Is My Health Data Safe?

Your health data, from daily steps to DNA, is sensitive and deserves protection. AI tools can enhance your health, but you must ensure your data stays secure. Reputable health AI companies use bank-level encryption to safeguard your information, making it unreadable without special keys. Laws like HIPAA in the U.S. set strict standards to prevent unauthorized sharing. To stay safe, always review an app's privacy policy before use, and consider tools that process data locally on your device. (Detailed privacy steps are in Appendix C.)

### Who Might Want Your Health Data?

Despite scary headlines, most people's health data isn't very valuable to bad actors. They are more interested in your financial information. Here's who might be interested in your health information and why:

**Marketers and Advertisers:** Companies might want to target you with products based on your health status. While this might be annoying, it's rarely harmful. The Network Advertising Initiative says they need your clear consent for health-related ads anyway.

**Insurance Companies:** Health insurers already have access to your claims data. In the U.S., the Affordable Care Act stops them from denying coverage based on preexisting conditions. For life and disability insurance, companies can already require medical exams before coverage. So AI data don't create much in the way of new risks here.

**Employers:** HIPAA and the Americans with Disabilities Act provide strong legal protection. These laws make it illegal for employers to access your health information without your consent. They also can't discriminate based on health conditions.

**Hackers:** Hackers would rather get your credit card number than your step count. The Department of Health and Human Services reported 45 million health records affected by breaches in 2021, mostly from large hospital systems, not fitness apps. While alarming, the vast majority of people whose records were breached never experienced harm beyond the stress of being notified—hackers usually focus on financial information or passwords they can quickly turn into money.

**Government Agencies:** In democratic countries, government agencies usually need legal permission like a warrant to access private health data. These requests are usually targeted at specific people under investigation rather than mass watching of health records.

While foreign state actors do have clever and sneaky ways of accessing data, they generally focus these resources on high-value targets. This includes government officials, military personnel, and people with access to sensitive information—not the average person's health records. If you work in a sensitive position or have specific concerns about foreign watching, you might choose to be more careful with digital health tools. But for most people, this particular risk is small compared to the health benefits these tools provide.

### Legal Protections Continue Growing Stronger

The legal framework protecting your information continues to get stronger. HIPAA protects information shared with doctors and insurers. It sets rules for how your health data can be used and shared. The Federal Trade Commission can punish apps with poor security practices.

As we will explain in Chapter 2, the Genetic Information Nondiscrimination Act (GINA) protects your genetic information from most discrimination. But remember those important exceptions: life, disability, and long-term care insurance aren't covered by this law.

Before getting genetic testing, think about your insurance situation. If you might need life or long-term care insurance in the future, consider getting those policies first. Once you have genetic test results showing high risk for certain conditions, these insurers could charge you more or turn you down.

This doesn't mean you should avoid genetic testing. Most people won't have problems with their job or health insurance—GINA protects those. The key is planning ahead. Talk to a genetic counselor about what your results mean for your health. An insurance advisor can help you understand your coverage options before you test.

Your genetic information is powerful and personal. With the right planning, you can learn from your genes while still protecting yourself financially. Just take the simple step of checking your insurance needs before you spit in that tube.

The California Consumer Privacy Act and similar state laws give residents rights: They have the right to know what personal information companies collect, delete their data, and opt out of data sales. The European Union's General Data Protection Regulation provides even stronger protections for citizens of EU countries. According to the United Nations Conference on Trade and Development, over 71% of countries now have privacy laws. So this protective network is expanding globally.

### Different Communities, Different Concerns

Different groups have varying concerns about data privacy. This is based on past experiences and cultural factors. These views deserve not just recognition but genuine respect. They're based on very real past wrongs.

Black Americans often worry about sharing health data because of past harm done by the medical system. The Tuskegee study is one terrible example: for decades, doctors let Black men with syphilis go untreated just to see what would happen to them. This history of abuse still affects trust today. A 2020 survey found that 70% of Black adults believe the healthcare system treats people unfairly based on race, compared to only 41% of White adults (Kaiser Family Foundation & The Undefeated, 2020). These trust issues run deep—when medical systems have hurt your community before, you're more careful about sharing any kind of health information, whether with doctors or apps.

Hispanic communities sometimes worry about potential immigration implications of health data sharing. While Homeland Security has policies against using health data for immigration enforcement, past instances where supposed firewalls between systems were breached have created lasting wariness. For undocumented individuals or mixed-status families, these concerns can significantly impact healthcare decisions.

American Indian groups recall past research violations involving DNA studies. One example is with the Havasupai tribe. Blood samples collected for diabetes research were used without consent for unrelated studies on mental illness and population migration. Many tribal nations now maintain oversight of research and data collection affecting their communities.

Asian Americans generally align with overall population concerns. But they may be more reluctant to share information about potentially stigmatized conditions. This is due to cultural factors around privacy and family reputation.

Different communities' views on data privacy aren't problems to solve—they're valuable for building better systems. When health AI developers incorporate diverse viewpoints during development, their applications are better understood and more likely to be used (Reddy et al., 2020).

The medical field increasingly recognizes this need. Health technology developers have started to address cultural concerns in their privacy approaches and to document how different communities were involved throughout the development process (American Medical Association, 2024).

## Life-Changing Benefits Make It Worth It

Sharing health data with AI tools can greatly improve your well-being. In this book, we'll explore examples of how these technologies enhance healthcare, addressing both everyday and critical needs.

After Anthony's wife was diagnosed with breast cancer, AI gave detailed guidance on treatment options. It suggested specific expert doctors by name. It found which medical centers offered the most advanced care for her cancer. This information proved very valuable during an overwhelming time when making the right treatment decisions quickly was crucial.

For Elena, who had been tracking her blood pressure readings for months without noticing any patterns, sharing this data with an AI analysis tool was like "the lights suddenly coming on in a dark room." The AI found that her blood pressure consistently spiked after certain foods and during specific times of day. These were insights her human doctor hadn't spotted in the same data.

Beyond personal stories, research backs up these benefits. AI can spot heart problems by reading ECG data—the same heart rhythm information that many smartwatches now collect (Attia et al., 2019). This technology finds heart issues before people feel sick, which could save lives by catching problems early.

For people with long-term health conditions, AI tools help track daily symptoms, how medicines are working, and whether the condition is getting better or worse. This leads to better care and a better life. For example, AI tools that help manage diabetes can prevent serious problems and help people keep their blood sugar at healthy levels (Ellahham, 2020).

AI tools can make healthcare work better during emergencies by helping doctors monitor patients from far away (Reddy et al., 2019). When COVID-19 hit, these tools became even more important. They let doctors check on sick people through video calls and track their health without risky in-person visits. This kept vulnerable patients safe while still getting them the care they needed. The pandemic proved how valuable AI can be for keeping healthcare running when people can't safely visit doctors' offices.

## Working With Your Doctor in the AI Age: Trust But Verify

The relationship between a patient and their doctor is like a carefully planned dance. It's a partnership built on trust, expertise, and shared goals. Yet, like any dance, it has its challenges. In emergencies, a doctor's training and judgment are invaluable. When you're rushed to the ER with chest pain, there's no time for second-guessing. In these critical moments, trust in your doctor's ability to act swiftly can mean the difference between life and death.

But outside of life-threatening scenarios, the dance becomes more complex. Doctors, for all their knowledge and professionalism, are human. They work under huge time constraints and packed schedules that don't always allow for in-depth conversations. They can make mistakes—not usually from carelessness, but because medicine is constantly evolving, and every patient is different.

This means that in nonemergency situations, you should take an active role in your own care. The best approach is to engage as an informed participant. Trust in your doctor's expertise while also taking responsibility for understanding your options and making decisions that align with your health goals.

One valuable tool for an informed patient is a second opinion, especially for elective procedures. Unlike emergency surgeries, elective procedures allow time for reflection and research. This includes things like knee replacements or most spinal surgeries. While a doctor may confidently recommend a procedure, another specialist might suggest alternative treatments that could be equally effective with fewer risks.

Seeking a second opinion isn't an act of distrust. It's a way to ensure all options are considered. Most doctors encourage it because an informed patient is a better decision-maker. If your doctor reacts defensively to a second-opinion request, it may be a red flag.

## Using AI as a Bridge to Better Care

AI enhances your doctor visits by organizing health data for better discussions, but final diagnoses and treatments rely on your doctor's expertise. You're bringing more organized, meaningful information to the conversation. For example, if you've been tracking your sleep patterns with a wearable device, and AI analysis shows a link between poor sleep and certain behaviors, you can share this with your doctor. This data gives them valuable insights they wouldn't otherwise have. This allows for more personalized care.

Earlier, I mentioned asking AI for references to verify its claims. But AI can also help you research health topics more deeply. If AI suggests that certain symptoms might indicate a particular condition, ask it to find medical articles about it. You can read these articles yourself, or—since they can be technical—upload the PDF to AI and ask for a plain-language summary. This helps you understand your health concerns better and prepares you for more meaningful conversations with your doctor.

One area where AI can be particularly helpful is considering rare diseases. Doctors sometimes develop tunnel vision, focusing only on the most common conditions that match your symptoms. AI, on the other hand, keeps an open mind and can suggest uncommon possibilities that might otherwise be overlooked. This doesn't mean AI will always be right—it just means it can bring up conditions your doctor might want to consider.

### Finding Balance in Healthcare Partnerships

Here's how to navigate this partnership effectively:

- Trust your doctor in emergencies: Their expertise is critical in life-threatening situations.
- Be an active participant in nonemergency care: Ask questions, discuss options, and make sure you understand treatment plans.
- Seek second opinions for elective procedures: Different doctors may offer different approaches. Having more perspectives can help you make the best choice.
- Use AI as a research tool, not a final authority: AI can provide insights, but it doesn't replace a doctor's judgment.
- Ensure communication between specialists and primary doctors: Keep records and make sure all your doctors are aware of each other's recommendations.

The goal isn't to replace doctors with AI or second-guess every decision. It's to work together toward the best possible outcome.

By understanding your role, asking the right questions, and using tools like AI, you can take control of your health while maintaining a strong partnership with your medical team.

When it comes to making a final diagnosis and starting treatment, doctors still outshine AI. Doctors consider many factors that AI might miss—your full medical history, subtle physical exam findings, family dynamics, and the way you describe your symptoms or react during the visit. While AI can suggest possibilities, the final decision rests with you and your doctor working together. Your physician's medical opinion is still the most important one, and it's usually wise to follow their guidance on diagnosis and treatment plans.

## What You'll Learn in This Book

You'll learn a new trick: tell AI your health goals, and it crafts the perfect questions for you to ask AI—a "flipping the script" method that makes AI easy, even for beginners. You'll see real AI answers, including supplement suggestions, so it will become easier to use AI. Since health tech moves fast, we'll share questions to ask AI for the latest tools, keeping you up to date.

The book is divided into three main parts:

**Part 1: Reading Your Body's Signals** You'll learn how to choose the best wearable devices and apps for your health like heart health, sleep, or energy levels. We'll show you how to use AI to read the data from these tools so you can focus on what really matters without getting lost in numbers. We'll also explain how AI helps make genetic test results easier to understand and act on. You'll learn how to choose the right tests, understand the results, and talk with your doctor about what they mean.

**Part 2: Smart Health Solutions** This section covers how AI can help you stay ahead of major health problems, such as heart disease, memory loss, diabetes, and weight management.

You'll learn how AI can find early warning signs—giving you and your doctor time to act. We'll also talk about stroke prevention, early cancer detection, depression, and how to protect your lungs.

**Part 3: Personalized Prevention** You'll learn how to talk to your doctor about using AI and how to safely use it for things like choosing supplements, avoiding drug interactions, and improving your health routines. For example, one of my patients—let's call her Julia—used an app that warned her about a dangerous drug interaction that her doctors had missed.

**Special Focus Areas** You don't need to be tech-savvy to use this book. It includes easy-to-follow steps and helpful tips in case anything feels confusing, like how to upload your data.

We'll also explore how AI can help you live longer—and better. You'll learn about science-backed tools that may support your cells and slow aging. These are things you can start using today.

We'll end with a look at the future of health technology. You'll learn what's already available and what's still being developed—so you're ready for what's next.

**A Different Kind of Health Book** Most health tech books either confuse readers with too much technical language or make big promises they can't keep. *Better Health with AI* is different. It uses clear language and realistic examples to show how AI can support your health.

This book also talks about when AI doesn't work and what to do when the healthcare system falls short. For example, AI helped my patient Lisa improve her energy within a week by suggesting a 10-minute morning walk after noticing that her afternoon energy crashed. Always choose apps with encryption to keep your data safe, ensuring you can confidently use these tools. You'll learn when to trust AI and when to turn to human experts.

Above all, this book is about giving you more control. Whether you're living with a health problem, trying to avoid one, or just want to feel your best, AI can help—if you use it wisely and with guidance.

Ready to take control of your health with AI? Let's begin.

# PART 1:

## Reading Your Body's Signals

CHAPTER 1

# THE HEALTH DIARY ON YOUR WRIST

As I researched this book, I discovered something unexpected: The most revealing health data isn't just in medical charts. It's being collected right now, all around us.

That smartphone in your pocket is remarkably powerful—more than the computers that sent astronauts to the moon. But here's what might surprise you more: it's already equipped with health sensors that can track your vital signs. Nearly 90% of Americans carry this health monitoring tool every day without realizing all it can do.

Your smartphone has motion sensors that count your steps by detecting the rhythm of walking. When you keep it near your bed, it can hear breathing patterns and small movements to estimate your sleep cycles. The phone is also smart enough to tell when you've fallen versus when it's just been dropped—when you fall, the phone detects the specific combination of sudden downward movement followed by no motion (because you're hurt) plus the horizontal position (you're lying down). When you just drop your phone, it hits the ground but then stays still in whatever position it lands. Amazingly, a phone can tell the difference and will try to call for help if it thinks you've fallen and aren't moving.

According to the 2023 Rock Health Digital Health Consumer Adoption Survey, 44% of Americans own wearable health tracking devices like smartwatches or smart rings (Rock Health, 2024). These wearables can do much more than phones. They track your heart rate all day, automatically measure blood oxygen levels, and monitor stress. They also track sleep better than phones because you wear them at night.

Your smartphone acts like a control center. It connects with your wearable to show and organize all this health data in apps like Apple Health or Google Fit. Together, they give you ongoing health information that helps you make smart decisions with your doctor.

When you share this combined data with AI tools, you get even deeper insights. AI can spot patterns across both devices. It might find irregular heart rhythms or gradually worsening sleep quality over weeks that you would miss on your own.

But most people never use this information to improve their health or don't use it to its fullest. They don't realize that their smartphones already contain free health apps they've never opened. Apple Health and Google Fit come preinstalled on most phones, quietly collecting basic data waiting to be used. Beyond these, many other health apps can make your smartphone better at tracking health. Popular ones include MyFitnessPal for food tracking, Sleep Cycle for better sleep monitoring, and Headspace for stress management. Many are free or cheap, and you don't need to buy extra devices.

Others with more capabilities are modest in cost. For example, HeartWatch ($4.99) provides deeper insights into heart rate patterns. Sleep Cycle ($39.99/year) analyzes your sleep patterns and wakes you at the best possible time. You set your alarm for, say, 7:00 AM, and the app monitors you during the 30 minutes before that. When it detects you're in light sleep—instead of deep sleep—it wakes you then. This helps you feel refreshed rather than groggy, even if it means waking a few minutes early. Even the premium services like Oura ($5.99/month) offer free trials so you can determine whether the extra features are worth the cost for your needs. Ask a large language model (LLM) AI app, such as Grok, Claude, Gemini, or ChatGPT for phone fitness apps and wearables, as this is a quickly growing field.

The best thing about this data is that it's continuous and current. While lab results provide occasional snapshots of your health, phones and wearables track important health information every minute of every day.

Research shows these devices track sleep patterns very well. They're less than 10% different from hospital sleep tests. They work as early warning systems. They spot patterns you should discuss with your doctor.

Starting with AI for health is very simple—you can begin if you have a smartphone already in your pocket. Learn to open your phone's health app, explore its features, and consider adding specialized apps based on your health priorities. The key isn't having the most expensive wearable but consistently using whatever tools you have, even if it's just your smartphone and a free app that helps you track how you feel each day.

## What Your Wearable Actually Tracks

Your wearable device collects more health information than you might expect. It doesn't just measure your heart rate now. It monitors your patterns all day and night. This shows how your body handles activities and stress. These devices divide your sleep into parts. They show time spent in light sleep, deep sleep, and dream sleep (REM). This information helps you understand how well you rest. A tiny sensor inside follows your movements in all directions. It counts your steps and calories used. It works whether you're walking slowly or exercising hard.

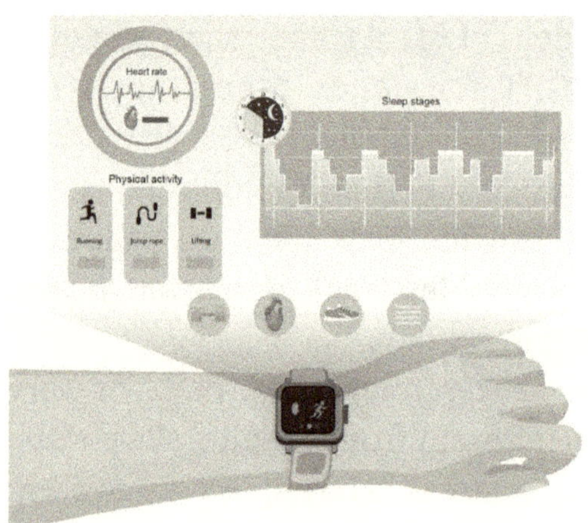


AI-based wearable devices can continuously collect health data such as heartbeat rate, sleep quality, and level of physical activity, indicating small yet unnoticeable variations in these values

Heart rate variability (HRV) is a key feature. This measures the tiny changes in time between your heartbeats. Even though your heart might beat 60 times per minute, those beats aren't perfectly spaced—one gap might be 1.01 seconds, the next 0.98 seconds, then 1.02 seconds. These small variations show your stress and recovery levels. These changes are actually good—they show your heart can adjust quickly to what your body needs. Higher HRV usually means better heart health and that you're managing stress well. Low HRV might mean you need more rest.

Newer devices measure your blood oxygen—how much oxygen is in your blood. Some also check temperature changes through your wrist or finger. These measurements, analyzed by AI on your phone, can catch early illness signs before you feel sick.

### What Your Wearable Doesn't Track... Yet!

It's equally important to understand current limitations:

- Blood pressure and blood sugar still require separate devices.
- Mental health metrics are limited and indirect.
    - Wearables can track sleep HRV, resting heart rate, physical activity, and skin temperature, which may correlate with stress, anxiety, or depressive states.
    - However, they cannot diagnose depression or anxiety, and changes in metrics (like walking fewer steps) are nonspecific.
- These devices cannot diagnose medical conditions—only suggest when to seek professional evaluation.

As wearable technology advances rapidly, you can use an AI assistant to check current capabilities. Simply ask: "What health metrics can be tracked and by which devices?" This will give you the most up-to-date information about your specific device's features.

### Recognizing Health Apps on Your Devices

Wondering which health apps to find on your phone or wearable? They have clear, easy-to-spot icons. Apple Health has a white square with a red heart symbol on iPhones. Samsung Health shows a white heart on a pink or red background. Google Fit features a colorful heart design with blue and yellow sections on Android phones.

Since new health apps come out regularly, you can ask an AI assistant for a current list. Try asking: "What are the most common health apps and what do their icons look like?"

### A Real-World Example: Detecting Heart Rhythm Problems Before a Stroke

Here's how wearables can save your life. Atrial fibrillation (AFib) is an uneven heartbeat—much beyond the micro-differences that HRV measures. It affects over 6 million Americans and increases stroke risk. AFib is dangerous because it often has no signs. Many don't know they have AFib until a stroke hits. An uneven heartbeat lets blood collect in the heart. This creates clots that may reach the brain. People with AFib are five times more likely to have a stroke.

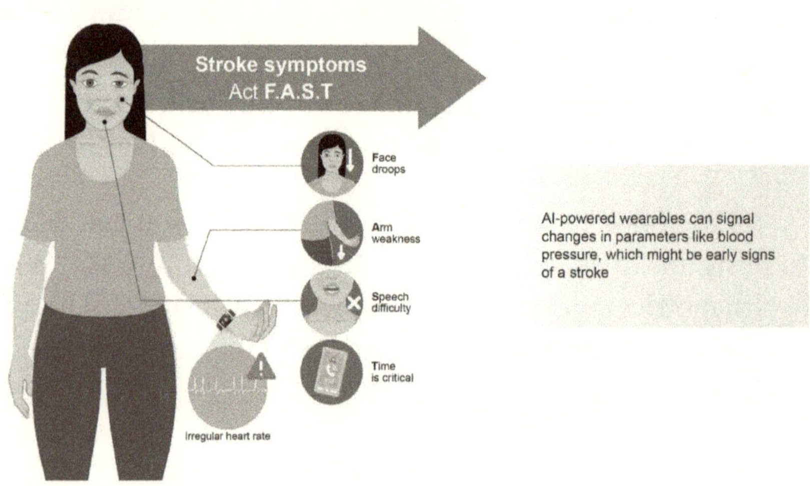

Stroke symptoms
Act F.A.S.T
Face droops
Arm weakness
Speech difficulty
Time is critical
Irregular heart rate
AI-powered wearables can signal changes in parameters like blood pressure, which might be early signs of a stroke

This is where your wearable device and AI can make a life-saving difference. Your device might spot warning signs before you notice anything. It might find irregular heart rhythms during rest or sleep. It could catch sudden heart rate jumps when you're not active. It might see unusual patterns in how your heart beats. Or it could find times when your heart rate goes over 110 beats per minute while you're resting (normal is 60–80 bpm). These subtle signals are invisible to you, but your wearable catches them.

AI can now detect AFib in remarkable ways. Even when your heart rhythm looks completely normal during an EKG, AI can spot subtle patterns that show you have AFib at other times (Attia et al., 2019). It's like your heart leaves invisible "fingerprints" of AFib that only AI can see—tiny changes in the electrical waves that are too subtle for doctors to notice.

This matters because AFib often comes and goes, making it hard to catch during a regular doctor's visit. You might have AFib several times a week, but if it's not happening during your 15-minute appointment, a standard EKG would miss it. Finding AFib early is crucial—treatment with blood-thinning medications reduces stroke risk by about 64% (Hart et al., 2007). That's why this AI technology is so exciting: it can identify a serious condition even when it's playing hide-and-seek.

Robert, a 61-year-old accountant, got an Apple Watch for his birthday. Three weeks later, it warned him about an irregular heart rhythm. He felt fine and almost ignored it. But his wife made him call his doctor. A heart test confirmed AFib. "I had no idea anything was wrong," Robert said. "That watch notification probably prevented a stroke. Now I'm on the right medication because my watch caught something I couldn't feel."

### Beyond AFib: Other Health Patterns Wearables Can Reveal

Your wearable can catch health issues beyond irregular heartbeats, giving you early warnings to act on:

**Trouble breathing at night?** Your wearable tracks oxygen levels while you sleep. Low oxygen might indicate sleep apnea, a medical problem that causes your breathing to stop for 10–30 seconds or longer while you sleep. Many people don't realize they have it. It can cause cardiovascular problems, daytime fatigue and cognitive issues, mental health challenges, type 2 diabetes, weight gain and obesity, weakened immune function, liver dysfunction, and a decreased quality of life. Talk to your doctor if your data shows anything unusual—whether it's oxygen drops below 90%, frequent breathing interruptions, or other abnormal patterns.

**Feeling fine but getting sick?** Your wearable might notice a slight fever or heart rate change days before symptoms hit. Research shows wearables can detect illness signs 1–2 days before symptoms appear. Ask your AI app to track these trends. Flu medicines work very well when you start them early (Dobson et al., 2015). Similarly, taking vitamin C when you first get cold symptoms can shorten how long you're sick (Hemilä & Chalker, 2013).

**Stress affecting your heart?** Your wearable tracks heart rate changes when you're stressed. Constant stress can raise blood pressure over time. Try a meditation app if your HRV drops below 20 milliseconds for a week. If that doesn't work, consider seeing a professional.

**Recovering from illness or surgery?** Your wearable tracks heart rate, sleep, and activity to show how you're healing. For example, steady HRV improvement means you're on track. Share recovery trends with your doctor.

**Struggling with exercise?** If your heart rate jumps too high during light activity, like over 120 bpm on a walk, it might hint at heart or lung issues. Check with your doctor if this happens often. Whoop recently added a new feature called Advanced Labs that shows how fitness trackers are becoming complete health tools. You can upload blood test results from your doctor for free, or pay for new blood tests through the app ($199 for one test, $349 for two annually, or $599 for four). What's special is how Whoop connects your blood test results to your daily tracking data. The AI looks at 65 different blood markers and figures out how they relate to your sleep, heart rate, and exercise data. Then a doctor reviews everything and creates a personal plan that shows up right in your app. For example, if your blood shows high inflammation, the AI might notice you've been sleeping poorly and suggest eating different foods or exercising less intensely. This creates a loop where your blood tests help guide what you do every day. While other wearable companies are exploring similar features, this deep integration of blood testing with daily tracking represents the future of personalized health monitoring.

These patterns warn you and your doctor about health issues early. Focus on trends over weeks, not one-time readings.

### The Challenge: Getting Your Data to Work for You

Your wearable tracks thousands of health measurements, but here's the problem: that data just sits there. Most devices don't automatically turn your numbers into useful health insights. You need to bridge the gap between collecting data and using it.

Think about Leslie, a teacher who felt tired for months. Her fitness tracker showed her sleep scores dropping week by week, but she didn't notice the pattern until her daughter helped her look at 3 months of data together. The trend was clear: her deep sleep had fallen by 30%. This insight led to a sleep study that found sleep apnea. Now she uses a CPAP machine and feels energetic again.

Here's how you can access your health story: Most health apps have an "Export" button in their settings menu. Look for words like "Export," "Share Data," or "Download." This creates a file you can review or share with your doctor. Apple Health users can tap "Browse," then your profile picture, then "Export All Health Data." For other devices, try asking an AI assistant: "How do I export my [device name] health data to review or share with my doctor?"

Not comfortable with technology? No problem. Take screenshots of important trends in your health app. Your doctor can work with pictures.

**Keep your data safe.** When sharing health information, choose apps with strong privacy settings. Look for apps that encrypt your data or let you control who sees it.

Your health data tells a story. The key is learning how to read it and share it safely with people who can help you stay healthy.

## Three Simple Steps to Start Using Your Data Today

To start using your health data, choose one thing to track, like sleep quality. Check weekly trends, not daily numbers, to see true changes. If you see worrying trends, jot them down for your doctor's visit.

Here's an easy way: Write daily how you feel next to what your app, like Apple Health, shows. Even without fancy AI, you can find clues. For example, tracking mood in Apple Health showed Jane had more energy after morning walks.

## My Journey, Your Mirror

Besides developing AI approaches for health, I'm no tech expert. Those activity rings on my watch? For years, I ignored them until I spent a few minutes checking what they tracked. The clues were there all along—I just had to look.

Many of you wear health trackers too. They've become a big part of my daily life. I found that too much morning iced green tea or occasional diet cola keeps me up at night. I write best at 5 a.m. after 7–8 hours of good sleep. Overdoing late walks or golf keeps my heart rate up at night, making me feel tired the next day—my Oura Ring shows this with a lower readiness score.

Like me, you can find helpful insights about your sleep, exercise, stress, or even early health warnings. Wearables and AI can change how you understand your body.

Don't obsess over every number—just look for clues you might miss. Your wrist holds health data waiting for you to explore. The next chapter shows how to use these numbers to boost your health, not just to spark curiosity. Tech-savvy or not, I'll share easy ways to turn data into health tips you can use. Check your app's summary screen today to start.

Curious about what your wearable can show you? Ready to learn how to use it smartly?

## Key Takeaways

Here's what matters most: Wearables watch your health all the time and can spot changes before you feel sick. They help your doctor but don't replace checkups. Start simple—pick one thing to track and look for weekly patterns. Share any worrying trends with your doctor. Remember, when it comes to your health, being good most of the time beats being perfect sometimes.

CHAPTER 2

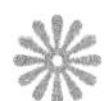

# AI MAKES YOUR GENES EASY TO UNDERSTAND

Getting a genetic test result can feel like receiving a letter in a secret code. Your DNA, the instructions that make you unique, is stored in a file with a long string of letters: A, T, G, and C—names for chemicals in your DNA. These are the building blocks of your genes.

You have about 22,000 genes. No wonder we need AI! This chapter discusses just four important genes as examples: apolipoprotein E *(APOE*—brain health and cholesterol metabolism), *BRCA1/BRCA2* (DNA repair and cancer prevention), *MTHFR* (folate processing and medication metabolism), and 9p21 (cardiovascular disease risk regulation).

Tools like ChatGPT, Claude, Gemini, and Grok can't read DNA code directly—it's like trying to bake a fancy cake in a microwave; it just doesn't work. These tools aren't built to decode those letters. Instead, these AI tools shine when they take your genetic test report—a summary created by a lab—and explain it in simple words.

Behind the scenes, professional labs use specialized AI programs to turn your raw genetic data into useful information. Companies like Illumina, Pacific Biosciences, and Oxford Nanopore use AI-powered tools to read and interpret the millions of DNA letters in your genome. These professional systems do the heavy lifting—converting all those A's, T's, G's, and C's into a report that actually means something. Then consumer AI can help you understand what that report says about your health.

They can also suggest practical steps to take. For example, if a test from a company like AncestryDNA says, "Your *APOE* gene is ε3/ε4," you might wonder what that means. You can ask an AI tool: "What does *APOE* ε3/ε4 mean, and what should I do about it?" Let's explore how AI can help you understand this kind of result. Here's how Grok might explain an *APOE* ε3/ε4 result:

The *APOE* gene helps your body manage cholesterol and keep your brain healthy. This gene comes in three types: *APOE* ε2, *APOE* ε3, and *APOE* ε4. You inherit one copy from your mom and one from your dad, so you have two copies. *APOE* ε2 is rare and protects people from heart and brain diseases. *APOE* ε3 is the most common version and doesn't increase your risk for diseases. *APOE* ε4, however, can raise your chances of developing Alzheimer's disease or heart problems later in life. If you have *APOE* ε3/ε4, you have one copy of each version. This means you have about a 25% chance of getting Alzheimer's by age 85, compared to a 12% chance for most people (Norwitz et al., 2021).

But many people with one or two copies of *APOE* ε4 never develop Alzheimer's. Things like your diet, exercise, and other genes play a big role. *APOE* ε4 might also slightly increase your risk of heart problems, especially if you don't eat healthily or stay active.

What should you do with this information? It might seem overwhelming at first. If it's hard to understand, you can tell the AI: "Make it simpler" or "Make it shorter and easier," and it will rephrase the explanation.

Start by telling your doctor about your *APOE* ε3/ε4 result. Ask for a checkup to measure your cholesterol and blood pressure. If you're feeling worried, a genetic counselor, who is an expert in explaining DNA results, can help.

You can lower your risks a lot by making healthy choices, even if you have *APOE* ε4 (Livingston et al., 2024). Try a Mediterranean diet with lots of vegetables, fruits, fish, and nuts, and eat less red meat and fewer sugary foods.

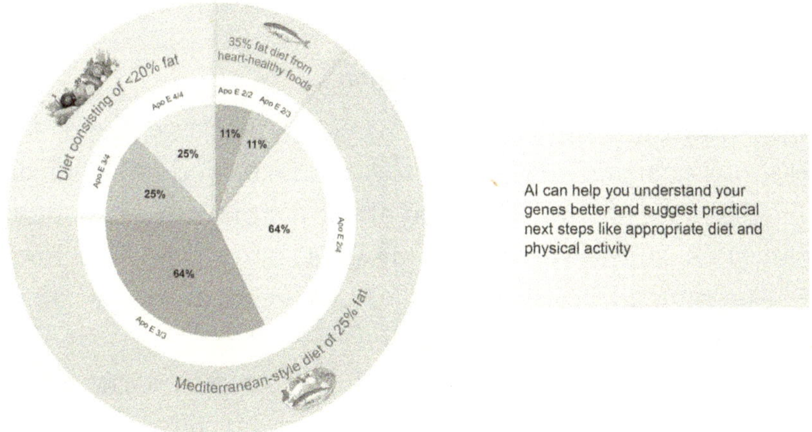


Exercise for at least 150 minutes each week, such as walking or biking. Sleep 7–9 hours every night. Keep your brain active by reading, solving puzzles, or learning something new. Manage stress with activities like meditation or deep breathing.

Check your cholesterol and blood pressure regularly to keep your heart healthy. Don't smoke, and if you drink alcohol, limit it to one or two drinks, and not every day. Stay at a healthy weight and spend time with friends and family, as social connections help your brain.

Avoid unproven supplements or products claiming to be "miracle cures." If you notice memory problems or have family members with Alzheimer's, ask your doctor about memory tests.

If you're nervous, a genetic counselor can clarify your results. Don't overthink your *APOE* ε3/ε4 result—it raises risk but doesn't guarantee illness. Genetic data, like *BRCA* results, is sensitive. Laws like GINA limit employer or insurer misuse, but choose apps with encryption and user-controlled sharing to protect it. (See Appendix C for safe data-sharing tips.) Your health data is a powerful tool when shared securely with your doctor.

### How AI Simplifies Genetic Information

Now that you understand how AI explains a gene like *APOE*, let's look at how it helps with other genes. Genetic tests look at specific parts of your DNA that affect your health. A lab turns your DNA sample (usually from saliva) into a report. AI takes that report and explains it in clear, everyday words, suggesting steps based on science.

For example, the *BRCA1* and *BRCA2* genes can affect your risk of breast cancer. These genes can have thousands of changes, called variants (abnormal genes). Some variants increase breast cancer risk, especially before age 70, while others are harmless. AI can explain what your specific variant means (Daly et al., 2023).

If you're curious about how this works, AI looks at your DNA like a recipe book, spotting small changes that might affect how your body follows the instructions. For example, in the *BRCA* genes, some changes make it harder for your cells to fix damaged DNA, which is why they raise cancer risk. But remember, this is just one piece of your health puzzle—your doctor can help put it all together.

Some variants are unclear, and AI can describe what's known about them. For instance, Jennifer used AI to understand her *BRCA2* variant, which led her to start mammograms earlier than typical and catch cancer early.

AI also helps with how your body handles medicines. Rebecca's test showed her *MTHFR* genes make her process some antidepressant medicines slowly. AI suggested she ask her doctor about medicines that might work better for her body (Klein et al., 2017).

The 9p21 gene variant increases heart attack risk. If you have it, AI recommends checking your blood for inflammation and talking to your doctor about heart health steps.

Tools like ChatGPT explain the well-known genes we have discussed. Companies like New Amsterdam Genomics use advanced and specialized AI to help generate your genetic reports. As you will see later in the book, AI has many roles in genetics as it does generally in medicine—helping the consumer, the lab, the doctor, and the researcher (Ho et al., 2020).

### Understanding the Limitations of Genetic Testing

While genetic testing offers valuable insights, it's important to understand its limitations and potential downsides. Genetic tests don't predict your future with certainty—they show probabilities, not guarantees. Many people with high-risk genetic variants never develop the associated conditions, while others without these variants still might.

Test results can cause unnecessary anxiety or false reassurance. Learning about increased disease risk when no proven prevention exists can be emotionally challenging. Conversely, having "low-risk" variants might lead to neglecting healthy lifestyle choices that benefit everyone regardless of genetics.

Privacy concerns are significant. Although there are legal protections like GINA, genetic information could potentially affect life insurance, employment, or family relationships. Data breaches at testing companies could expose sensitive information about you and your relatives who share your DNA.

Testing accuracy varies widely. While medical-grade tests are highly reliable, direct-to-consumer tests may miss important variants or provide incomplete information. Some tests analyze only common genetic changes, potentially missing rare but significant variants (Bean et al., 2021).

Additionally, genetic testing reveals information about your biological relatives who haven't consented to this disclosure. Family dynamics can be strained by unexpected discoveries about paternity, adoption, or disease risks that affect multiple family members.

Finally, the interpretation of genetic data is constantly evolving. A variant classified as harmless today might be reclassified as significant tomorrow, or vice versa, as scientific understanding advances.

## Exploring Genetic Testing Options

Before diving into specific tests, let's consider why you might want one. Genetic tests can tell you about your health risks or how your body works. They range from simple to advanced, and AI can help you decide if testing is right for you. You can start by asking AI about genes you're curious about—it's free and can guide your decision.

Basic tests like AncestryDNA ($99) focus on family history but let you download genetic data to check health information. MyHeritage DNA ($149) includes basic health reports. CircleDNA ($189) offers over 500 reports with AI insights.

More comprehensive options include Nebula Genomics ($299), with a chat feature to ask about your DNA, and Helix ($499), which looks at all 20,000+ genes and provides updates over time. For medical-grade testing, Invitae ($850) offers tests for specific health concerns.

Premium services like Nebula Deep ($999) sequence your entire DNA and include lifetime AI access, while New Amsterdam Genomics ($3,000) provides detailed analysis with genetic counseling.

If you already have raw DNA data, there are affordable analysis options. Genetic Genie offers free basic reports, Promethease ($12) compares your data to scientific studies, and SelfDecode ($97/year) gives AI-powered health advice.

Some specialized tests focus on medication responses. OneOme RightMed ($249) shows how your genes affect medicines, sorting them into green, yellow, or red categories. These tests are often covered by insurance, as genes impact 70–80% of medicines (Zanger & Schwab, 2013).

To update the information above, use this prompt in an LLM AI: "Provide an update on genetic testing services: AncestryDNA, MyHeritage DNA, CircleDNA, Nebula Genomics (including Deep), Helix, Invitae, New Amsterdam Genomics,

Genetic Genie, Promethease, SelfDecode, OneOme RightMed, and similar new tests. For each, list:

- Test type (e.g., ancestry, health, pharmacogenomics)
- Key features (e.g., AI-driven insights, report count, genetic counseling)
- Current price (note subscriptions or insurance coverage)
- How it addresses health risks like cardiovascular disease or obesity (linked to sleep apnea)
- Use reliable sources (e.g., company websites) to verify prices and features"

## Why Genetic Information Matters

Understanding your genes can feel like a lot to handle, but it's a tool for better health. For example, James was scared when his test showed a risk of heart disease. AI helped him see that his diet and exercise habits mattered more than his genes. Genes are like a weather forecast—they show a chance of something happening, not a guarantee. Knowing your genes helps you take smarter steps to stay healthy.

For instance, people with Lynch syndrome need colonoscopies every 2 years instead of every 5–10 years—AI can suggest this (Dominguez-Valentin et al., 2019). Those with *APOE4* might benefit from earlier memory tests. People with iron-overload genes should donate blood regularly—AI can explain how this works. If you have high cholesterol genes, early cholesterol checks are key. AI explains these conditions clearly.

### Your Plan for Using Genetic Information

To make the most of genetic tests, start with realistic expectations. AI can't read raw DNA files, but it's great for explaining reports. If you're curious about your family background or health, try an affordable test. Instead of trying to understand everything in your report, ask AI to review your results and identify the most important or actionable findings. These usually involve disease risks you can actually do something about or medications you might respond to differently. AI can help you zero in on what matters and skip the noise. Always share significant results with your doctor.

Genes are just one part of your health, alongside diet, exercise, and sleep. For privacy, don't share raw DNA files or personal details when using AI—just ask about general gene changes. AI makes your genetic information easier to understand. As it improves, AI might one day analyze entire DNA files, but it's already helpful now (Dias & Torkamani, 2019).

My patient Dayo said it well: "AI didn't predict my future. It showed me my genetic tendencies, so I can make better choices every day." Be curious but cautious. Combine genetic insights with data from fitness trackers, lab tests, and lifestyle habits, as explained in this book. See Appendix C for details on using genetic data with other health information for AI analysis. The next chapters will show you how to apply this knowledge to specific health conditions.

# PART 2

## Smart Health Solutions

CHAPTER 3

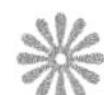

# HEART HEALTH AND AI: PARTNERS IN PREVENTION

Heart disease kills more people worldwide than anything else—about 18 million each year according to the World Health Organization (2024). While "heart disease" covers many conditions from irregular heartbeats to valve problems, coronary artery disease (CAD) is the deadliest kind. In the U.S. alone, it claims nearly 700,000 lives yearly.

Sarah's story demonstrates how technology can detect heart problems even when traditional symptoms aren't present. At 52, this marketing executive had always been active and had normal checkups, but her Apple Watch began showing concerning patterns in her HRV during her morning commute. "The app showed my HRV dropping significantly during my drive to work, even though I didn't feel particularly stressed," Sarah explains. Curious, she mentioned these patterns to her doctor, who recognized that reduced HRV can signal cardiovascular strain.

Despite Sarah having no chest pain or shortness of breath, her doctor ordered a CT coronary angiogram with HeartFlow analysis. While her calcium score was only moderately elevated, the AI-powered HeartFlow technology revealed what conventional imaging might have missed—a dangerous noncalcified "soft plaque," causing a 70% blockage in her left anterior descending artery, often called the widow-maker. This name is misleading since heart disease kills just as many women as men.

This discovery led to a minimally invasive procedure where cardiologists placed a drug-eluting stent (like a tiny spring) to open the artery and prevent a future heart attack. Sarah was also started on medications to lower cholesterol and prevent clotting.

"Without this AI analysis of my CT scan, they might have missed the soft plaque entirely until it was too late," Sarah reflects. "Thanks to the initial HRV data that prompted this advanced imaging, I'm back to my normal life with a much lower risk of having a heart attack." Stories like Sarah's are becoming more common—studies show that using AI to analyze heart scans catches dangerous blockages in about 20% more cases than traditional methods alone, potentially saving thousands of lives each year.

Sarah's case illustrates what makes heart disease so dangerous: how quietly it develops. About half of men and two-thirds of women who die suddenly from heart disease never noticed any symptoms. But AI tools are changing this by offering early warnings that our bodies—and even standard medical tests—might miss.

## Understanding Heart Disease

To understand how AI spotted Sarah's problem before symptoms appeared, it helps to know how heart disease develops. Here's something surprising: the heart itself often suffers from poor blood flow. Blood rushes through the heart constantly, but that's part of the problem—it moves too fast through the heart's chambers to feed the heart muscle. The heart's own cells depend on a separate blood supply system: coronary arteries that run along and through the heart muscle.

These coronary arteries face unique challenges. They're relatively small, and each one feeds a specific area of the heart without backup. If one gets blocked, blood flow stops immediately downstream. Within minutes, heart muscle cells start dying from lack of oxygen and sugar (glucose). After just a couple of hours without emergency treatment, the damage becomes permanent—what we call a heart attack (myocardial infarction).

But what causes these dangerous blockages? Recent research has changed how we think about heart disease. We now know lifestyle factors play a central role, alongside genetics and physical differences in heart structure. Let's look at what drives heart disease:

## Lifestyle Factors: The Foundation of Heart Health

### What We Eat and Blood Sugar Effects

What we eat might be the most important changeable risk factor for heart disease. Added sugars and refined carbohydrates are particularly concerning because they cause dangerous spikes in blood sugar. Research shows these repeated sugar spikes often start the process of artery damage—even in people without diabetes.

You've probably heard about antioxidants and how they're supposed to be good for you. That's because they help fight something called oxidative stress, which damages your body. But it's much better to prevent this damage in the first place than to try to fix it later with antioxidants. When blood sugar rises quickly after meals, it creates this oxidative stress that damages the inner lining of your arteries, setting the stage for plaque buildup.

These spikes cause real harm over time, even in people whose blood sugar looks normal during fasting tests. The worst culprits are sugary drinks: sodas top the list, but fruit juices aren't much better, and what many people don't realize is that those "healthy" smoothies from popular chains often pack just as much sugar as a soda. Desserts obviously spike blood sugar, but so do "white foods," the refined starches that are just chains of sugar molecules strung together. Bread, white rice, potatoes, pasta, and of course sugar itself all cause rapid blood sugar rises that damage your arteries.

Research shows that eating and drinking too much added sugar increases blood pressure, inflammation, weight gain, diabetes, and fatty liver disease (Hu & Malik, 2010; DiNicolantonio & O'Keefe, 2017). All of these problems work together to raise your risk of heart attack and stroke—studies show that people who get more than 25% of their calories from added sugar have nearly triple the risk of dying from heart disease (Yang et al., 2014).

As the body becomes more resistant to insulin and moves toward type 2 diabetes, these harmful effects get worse. The body struggles to control blood sugar, leading to chronically high levels that speed up blood vessel damage. This explains why countries with high diabetes rates have more heart disease, even when cholesterol levels are lower. The damage isn't limited to diagnosed diabetes—these changes begin years earlier as insulin sensitivity gradually declines.

Many people with metabolic syndrome—a cluster of conditions including high blood pressure, high blood sugar, excess belly fat, and slightly abnormal cholesterol patterns—develop heart disease even though their "bad" LDL cholesterol isn't particularly high.

### Sleep: Your Heart's Recovery Time

Sleep quality and duration significantly impact heart health. Both too little sleep (less than 7 hours) and too much (more than 9 hours) link to higher heart disease risk. Poor sleep raises stress hormones, increases blood pressure, and promotes inflammation.

Sleep apnea is especially dangerous, affecting 50–60 million Americans but diagnosed in only about 10% of cases. This condition causes oxygen levels to drop repeatedly during the night, triggering the body's fight-or-flight response and increasing heart disease risk by 200–300%. While wearables cannot formally diagnose sleep apnea, they excel at detecting the disrupted sleep patterns and overnight oxygen fluctuations it causes. Seeing this pattern allows you to bring it to the attention of your doctor, who can then order the appropriate medical testing to confirm the condition and begin potentially life-saving treatment.

Sleep is truly the cornerstone of health—like the foundation that supports an entire building, quality sleep holds up every other aspect of your well-being. Without it, everything else becomes shaky. Research shows that poor sleep not only directly damages your heart but also sets off a chain of unhealthy choices.

When you don't get enough sleep, your brain's hunger signals go haywire the next day, making you crave sugary, fatty foods instead of healthier options (Greer et al., 2013; St-Onge et al., 2016). Studies have also found strong links between poor sleep patterns and diets high in sugar and fat—people who sleep poorly tend to eat worse overall (Grandner et al., 2013). You also feel too tired to exercise, creating a vicious cycle: poor sleep leads to bad food choices and skipped workouts, which then make your sleep even worse. Each part of the cycle feeds the next, making it harder and harder to break free.

### Physical Activity: Your Heart's Shield

Regular exercise provides powerful protection against heart disease, reducing risk by 30–50% through several mechanisms. Research published in *The Lancet* found that individuals who maintained consistent physical activity had significantly lower cardiovascular disease rates compared to their sedentary counterparts, with the most active groups showing these large risk reductions (Lear et al., 2017).

### Stress: The Silent Heart Threat

Chronic stress activates biological pathways that directly damage the cardiovascular system. It raises cortisol levels, increases blood pressure, promotes inflammation, and disrupts sleep—all contributing to heart disease. Stress also makes it harder to maintain heart-healthy behaviors like proper diet and regular exercise. Managing stress through techniques like meditation, deep breathing, and adequate sleep provides significant heart protection.

## Heart Disease Risks Across Different Communities

Heart disease affects different groups of people in different ways. Some communities face higher rates of heart problems because of many factors—from access to healthy food and safe places to exercise to healthcare availability and everyday stress. New AI tools are starting to help with these differences, though we still have a long way to go.

Black Americans have higher rates of heart disease than other groups. Nearly half of Black women (48%) and men (44%) have some form of heart disease. High blood pressure is also more common, affecting about 56% of Black adults compared to 48% of White adults, and it often starts earlier in life. Things like limited access to healthcare, fewer healthy food options in some neighborhoods, and stress from racism all play important roles. Devices like the Omron HeartGuide watch show promise by letting people track their blood pressure accurately throughout the day.

Hispanic and Latino communities face their own challenges. Diabetes affects about 12% of Hispanic adults—compared to 7% of non-Hispanic Whites. Many have limited health insurance, and language barriers can make getting care harder. Spanish-language apps like Azumio Glucose Buddy help by making blood sugar tracking easier, even without internet access. This helps manage one of the biggest risk factors for heart disease.

Asian Americans often develop heart problems differently than other groups. Their bodies may show signs of trouble at lower weights—a BMI of 23 can indicate risk for Asian individuals, while the standard threshold is 25 for others. New AI systems recognize these differences and adjust their risk calculations accordingly, catching problems that might otherwise be missed.

American Indian communities have the highest diabetes rates in the U.S.: about 14% of adults. Many live in remote areas with few healthcare facilities nearby. The Indian Health Service has worked with tribes to create culturally respectful AI tools that work even with limited internet connection, focusing on lifestyle changes that honor traditional practices.

Pacific Islander communities face some of the world's highest rates of obesity and diabetes, with some islands reporting diabetes rates over 40%. Limited healthcare resources and geographic isolation make getting care difficult. New telemedicine platforms with AI support are beginning to bridge these gaps, though technology limitations remain. Many Pacific Islanders have seen their traditional diets replaced by less healthy Western foods, contributing to these problems. The most effective solutions respect cultural practices while addressing modern health challenges.

While these AI tools show promise, technology alone can't solve all these problems. The best approaches combine advanced tools with community programs and culturally appropriate care that respects each group's unique needs.

## How Heart Disease Develops

### Inflammation: The Common Pathway

Closely linked to diet, stress, and sleep quality, chronic inflammation is now recognized as a fundamental driver of atherosclerosis (artery hardening). A major study (CANTOS trial–lead author, Ridker) found that reducing inflammation in your body—even without changing cholesterol—cuts heart attack risk by 15%. This proves that inflammation damages your arteries just as much as cholesterol does. Even seemingly unrelated issues like gum disease can increase heart risk by 19%, as bacteria from infected gums enter the bloodstream and increase overall inflammation.

### Other Major Risk Factors

Smoking remains one of the most harmful risk factors you can control. It damages blood vessels in multiple ways—harming their inner lining, creating harmful chemicals in your blood, and directly poisoning heart tissue. Even occasional social smoking significantly increases your risk.

High blood pressure hurts your artery walls by putting too much force on them—like a river slowly wearing away rocks to create a canyon. When this happens, the artery walls get thicker and harder as they try to protect themselves from the extra pressure, accelerating plaque buildup. Each 20-point increase in systolic blood pressure doubles your risk of dying from heart disease. This pressure creates entry points for inflammatory cells and fats, speeding up the damage.

Your genes play a big role in heart disease risk. One area of DNA (the 9p21 region), called the heart attack gene, makes people 20–40% more likely to get heart disease, no matter what other risk factors they have.

Some genetic differences also change how well heart medicines work. For example, one gene affects how well cholesterol drugs called statins work for you. Another gene controls how your body handles blood thinners like clopidogrel (Plavix)—about 3 out of 10 people have a genetic difference that makes this common medicine not work well for them.

Other genetic differences affect a substance called lipoprotein(a) in your blood. When levels of this substance are high because of your genes, it can lead to more plaque buildup in your arteries and make blood clots more likely.

While no longer considered the primary cause of coronary artery heart disease for most people, high "bad" LDL cholesterol still plays an important role in plaque development once artery damage has begun. Research consistently shows that lowering LDL significantly reduces heart attack and stroke risk. People born with genetically low LDL levels have dramatically lower heart disease risk throughout life. When

LDL is lowered significantly through medications or lifestyle changes, plaque can actually shrink and stabilize, making it less likely to rupture and cause a heart attack.

Individual differences in coronary artery anatomy, including vessel twisting and branching angles, can increase vulnerability to narrowing and reduced blood flow. These anatomical variations help explain why some individuals with similar risk profiles experience different outcomes.

Understanding plaque formation reveals why coronary artery disease is so dangerous. Unlike mineral deposits in old pipes, arterial plaque develops inside the artery walls—not just sticking to the inner surface. The artery is living tissue, and fatty substances infiltrate between its layers. This creates two types of plaque: hard plaque (measured by coronary calcium scoring) and soft plaque (measured by AI analysis of a CT). Soft plaque, which forms within the artery wall, poses the greatest danger because it can rupture suddenly, triggering a blood clot (atheroma) that blocks the artery.

Most doctors now know that heart disease happens for different reasons in different people. Some people get heart disease mainly from high cholesterol. Others get it from high blood sugar, poor sleep, or too much stress. Your genes and your daily habits work together to affect your risk. That's why doctors need to look at everything, not just one thing. AI can help you track all these different health factors. It also helps doctors find out which problems are biggest for you. This way, doctors can make a treatment plan that fits your specific needs.

## Starting Simple: First Steps Before AI

If you want to start getting healthier, here are three simple things to do before using any AI tools.

First, eat smaller portions. Take whatever you normally eat and cut it in half. You can eat the same food, just save half for later or the next day. Instead of one big meal, you're making it into two smaller ones.

Second, start walking every day. Even 10 minutes is fine to start. Wear comfortable shoes and walk a little farther each day—but stop right away if you have chest pain or trouble breathing.

Third, start tracking something. Use a piece of paper, your computer, or your phone to write down one thing each day. It could be how far you walked, how many minutes you walked, or your weight (measured without clothes in the morning after using the bathroom).

Don't worry about picking the "right" thing to track. It really doesn't matter at first. I mentioned the Hawthorne effect in the Introduction. Factory workers in a study worked harder when the lights got brighter. But they also worked harder when the lights got dimmer. The workers weren't responding to the light—they were responding to being watched and measured.

The same thing happens when we track our own health. Just writing something down makes us want to do better. We like to see our numbers improve. After a few weeks of tracking, you'll have lots of data. That's when AI can help you spot patterns you might miss on your own.

## How AI is Transforming Heart Care

AI offers powerful new ways to monitor, detect, and manage heart disease, particularly by tracking lifestyle factors that form the foundation of heart health. Unlike traditional approaches that rely on occasional doctor visits and basic tests, AI can combine multiple data sources to provide personalized insights and continuous monitoring.

## Beyond Cholesterol: Finding Heart Disease Before Symptoms

For decades, we've relied on cholesterol tests to predict heart risk, but this approach misses many at-risk patients. People often show normal cholesterol despite having significant plaque buildup, while others only learn of their heart disease after failing a treadmill stress test.

AI-enhanced imaging has changed this landscape. Advanced CT scans analyzed by AI can now directly measure both calcified and soft plaque in arteries, assess blood flow restrictions, and identify vulnerable regions before symptoms occur. This earlier detection allows for intervention when it's most effective, often through lifestyle changes rather than invasive procedures.

This shift in diagnosis has sparked a parallel shift in treatment. Instead of primarily focusing on dietary cholesterol (which research shows has limited impact for most people), attention is now turning to inflammation control and blood sugar management.

## Building Your Heart Health Baseline

The first step toward prevention is understanding your current heart health status, with special attention to lifestyle factors. Wearables like the Apple Watch or Oura Ring measure HRV (how well your body handles stress and recovers), sleep quality and duration, and physical activity levels. Home blood pressure monitors provide clinical-grade measurements you can track over time, while smart scales track weight and body composition.

Medical tests remain essential—standard blood work and imaging studies provide critical baseline information that AI systems can analyze for subtle patterns. Beyond standard lipid panels, consider asking your doctor about advanced testing for inflammation markers like high-sensitivity C-reactive protein (hs-CRP) and tests for lipoprotein(a) levels, especially if you have a family history of early heart disease.

### Pairing Data for Deeper Insights

As you become more comfortable with basic tracking, you can start looking for connections between different aspects of your health. One revealing pairing is your step count and sleep quality. The relationship is U-shaped: the more you walk, the better you sleep, except if you overdo it, walk too late in the day, or fail to take an occasional rest day.

An even more powerful pairing combines food tracking with blood sugar monitoring. Apps like MyFitnessPal, Cronometer, and Lose It make food tracking simple—just take a photo of your meal, and the app identifies the foods and calculates nutrients. When paired with a continuous glucose monitor (CGM) like the FreeStyle Libre or Dexcom G6, you can see exactly how different foods affect your body.

CGMs are one of the most helpful tools for tracking blood sugar. The sensor sits on your skin for about 2 weeks. It's the size of a dime with a tiny needle that goes just under your skin. The needle is thinner than a human hair—so thin you won't feel it going in or while wearing it. I've worn one myself before recommending it to patients, and I honestly forgot it was there. A plastic protective cap covers everything, held in place by strong medical adhesive. Each sensor costs around $50–75 for 2 weeks of monitoring. While insurance typically covers them for people with diabetes, others can buy them without a prescription at most pharmacies.

CGMs eliminate finger pricks and send data straight to your phone. AI analyzes this information to predict blood sugar spikes before they happen. The system can suggest specific changes—like choosing oats instead of a donut—that can improve blood sugar control by about 30% based on current research.

Eat what you normally eat, and you'll quickly see how it affects your blood sugar, allowing you to make changes on your own. People respond very differently to foods. For instance, I had a banana with breakfast every day from childhood until I discovered it single-handedly spiked my blood sugar to 150.

Once you've collected both your food data and glucose readings, you can download your data from both systems (look for "Export Data" in your food tracking app settings and in your CGM app) and then ask an AI assistant to analyze the connections using this prompt:

"I've been tracking my food intake with [app name] and my blood glucose with [CGM brand] for 2 weeks. I've attached both data exports. Could you analyze:

1. Which specific foods or meals cause my highest glucose spikes
2. What patterns you notice in how my glucose responds to different food combinations
3. The best meal timing and composition for my unique metabolism based on this data
4. Three specific, actionable changes I could make that would have the biggest impact on stabilizing my blood sugar"

### Heart Data in Action: Getting the Most from AI

When it comes to heart health, the right data paired with effective AI prompts can provide insights that might otherwise remain hidden. Here's how to prepare your heart-related information for AI analysis and get useful answers.

### Preparing Your Heart Data

Your wearable device collects valuable information about lifestyle factors, but making it AI-ready requires a few simple steps:

Most devices like Apple Watch, Fitbit, and Oura Ring allow you to export your heart rate, ECG readings, activity data, and sleep metrics. Look for "Export" or "Share" options in your device's app, usually under Settings or Account. Take photos of your lab results, particularly lipid panels and blood glucose readings. AI can extract numbers from these images, though for best results, you might type key values into a simple notes file: "Total Cholesterol: 185, LDL: 110, HDL: 55, Triglycerides: 90, Date: 5/1/25."

Keep a basic text note of any heart-related symptoms like chest discomfort, shortness of breath, or unusual fatigue. Include when they occur and what you were doing. A simple format works best: "May 3: Shortness of breath while climbing stairs, lasted about 2 minutes." Track stress levels and diet choices alongside these notes for more comprehensive analysis. Also create a simple list of heart medications with dosages and when you started taking them. These details help AI understand changes in your health metrics.

### Effective Heart Health Prompts

The way you ask questions dramatically affects the quality of AI's insights. Here are sample prompts that work well for heart health analysis:

For blood pressure trends: "I've attached my blood pressure readings from the past month. Can you identify any patterns related to time of day or day of week? Are there consistent spikes or drops that might warrant discussion with my doctor?"

For wearable heart rate data: "Looking at my attached heart rate data, are there any unusual patterns during sleep or exercise? How does my heart rate variability compare to typical ranges for my age and activity level?"

For medication effectiveness: "Based on my cholesterol levels before and after starting a statin [say which drug and how many milligrams], how does my response compare to typical results? Are there any patterns in my side effects notes that might be worth discussing with my doctor?"

Most importantly, AI can now generate personalized plans to minimize your heart disease risk by optimizing lifestyle factors. For an up-to-date, personalized AI-generated plan to prevent a heart attack, try asking an AI assistant about your specific situation, including your age, sex, family history, lifestyle factors, and existing conditions. It will analyze your specific risk factors and recommend which tests and data are needed based on your individual profile. Remember to verify AI recommendations with your healthcare provider before making significant health decisions.

Apps called data integration platforms can transform how you manage your heart health information by automatically combining lifestyle data from multiple devices and apps in one place. Services like Heads-Up Health bring together medical records, lab results, wearable data, and nutrition tracking into comprehensive dashboards. Other options include Cronometer for detailed nutrition and biometric tracking and HealthMatters for clinical-grade integration of home health devices.

### Prevention: Using AI to Stop Heart Disease Before It Starts

AI excels at finding subtle patterns in lifestyle data that precede disease development, potentially allowing for intervention years before symptoms appear. AI can analyze ongoing data from wearable devices—detecting abnormal heart responses to exercise, concerning trends in blood pressure, harmful glucose spikes after meals, and sleep disturbances linked to heart disease. It can also tailor guidance based on your specific risk profile, prioritizing what matters most for your particular combination of risk factors. AI systems now outperform traditional risk calculators that doctors have used for decades. A recent study showed a deep learning algorithm analyzing ECG data could identify future heart rhythm problems with much greater accuracy than standard methods.

Keisha, a 52-year-old teacher with a family history of heart disease, had normal blood pressure and cholesterol at checkups. But her Apple Watch detected declining HRV and irregular nighttime heart rhythms. "My doctor was surprised when I showed her the data," Keisha says. "She ordered tests that found early signs of heart muscle stiffening that we caught before any damage was done." The wearable also tracked her sleep quality, revealing frequent disruptions that were contributing to inflammation—information she used to prioritize better sleep habits as part of her prevention plan.

## AI Tools That Work Now

AI tools use wearables to monitor heart health. For example, Cardiogram ($0–14.99/month) detects irregular rhythms with 97% accuracy, while Lark Health ($20/month) coaches blood pressure management. Sleep tracking apps with AI analysis can identify patterns of disruption associated with higher heart risk, while nutrition apps can detect harmful eating patterns.

For deeper analysis, FDA-approved AI algorithms can spot two different things in standard ECGs. As mentioned earlier, they can detect if someone has atrial fibrillation even when their heart rhythm looks normal during the test—the AI sees subtle "fingerprints" that AFib leaves behind. They can also pick up tiny electrical changes that suggest the heart isn't getting enough blood flow, which often means blocked arteries. While the ECG can't actually show the blockages themselves, it can reveal their effects on the heart's electrical signals. Ask your doctor if they have access to this AI technology or could get it—don't be surprised if they're not familiar with it yet. Many doctors are just learning about these tools, and your question might encourage them to look into options that could benefit all their patients.

### Your Roadmap to Better Heart Health Through AI

Begin with basic monitoring tools focused on lifestyle factors that won't strain your budget or overwhelm you with complexity. Smartphone health apps can track basic information like steps, heart rate, and sleep, while free apps let you log diet choices and blood pressure readings. When you're ready for more objective data, consider a connected blood pressure monitor that syncs with your phone to track trends over time ($40–100). Basic fitness trackers ($50–150) add continuous heart rate and sleep tracking to build a more complete picture.

As you become more comfortable with these tools, you might explore more comprehensive options like advanced wearables with ECG capabilities ($150–400) or home ECG devices ($89–149). Some people find CGMs helpful for tracking blood sugar patterns, even without diabetes. These devices cost $150–300 per month, but you can learn a lot from wearing one for just 2 weeks for less than $100. They help you see which foods cause inflammation in your body.

Genetic testing gives you lifetime insights into your personal heart risk. You have several options depending on your budget and needs. Targeted panels look at specific heart-related genes ($200–500). Whole genome sequencing examines all your DNA—think of it like reading a book once versus reading it 30 or 100 times to catch every detail.

### What Does "30x" or "100x" Coverage Mean?

When a lab sequences your genome, they don't just read your DNA once. Think of it like reading a difficult handwritten letter—you'd probably read it several times to make sure you understood it correctly.

Here's how it works: The lab breaks your DNA into millions of tiny pieces, reads each piece, then uses computers to put them back together like a puzzle. The "x" number tells you how many times, on average, each spot in your DNA gets read.

- **30x coverage** means each spot gets read about 30 times. This catches most errors and costs less ($300–500).
- **100x coverage** means each spot gets read about 100 times. This is like having 100 factcheckers instead of 30—you can be much more confident about rare or unusual genetic changes that might be important for your health ($500–1,000).

For most people, 30x coverage provides reliable results. But if you have a strong family history of genetic conditions or you're making major medical decisions based on your results, 100x coverage gives you extra confidence that you're seeing real genetic changes, not testing errors.

For those wanting comprehensive support, premium services like New Amsterdam Genomics ($3,000+) include the most thorough testing plus ongoing access to genetic counselors and lifetime reanalysis as science advances. Any of these options helps you create smarter, more targeted prevention strategies.

Integration platforms can bring together information from multiple sources to identify patterns between lifestyle factors and heart health markers, while AI analysis tools help you understand what changes might be meaningful. Most importantly, share relevant findings with your healthcare provider, who can help you decide which measurements are most important for you.

## Looking Forward

AI is transforming heart care from reactive disease management to proactive prevention through continuous monitoring of lifestyle factors and early intervention. This shift is already happening through practical tools available today, and the integration is becoming more seamless every year.

Consider how the next generation of gut microbiome analysis, already beginning with companies like Genova and Viome, might detect inflammatory markers that signal increased heart risk long before traditional tests. Your digestive system serves as an early warning system for inflammation that affects your arteries.

Researchers are developing even simpler tests that could catch heart issues before you feel sick. AI analysis of breath compounds, being developed at centers like the Cleveland Clinic, may soon detect heart cell stress through simple breath tests you could perform at home. Advanced sleep monitoring may detect subtle breathing disruptions that impact heart health long before they progress to clinical sleep apnea.

The combination of genetic testing with continuous lifestyle monitoring is perhaps most promising. Imagine learning you carry the heart attack gene variant then having an AI system specifically tuned to watch for the earliest signs of the problems this gene typically causes—perhaps by monitoring specific inflammatory markers or subtle changes in blood sugar regulation. This personalized approach—tailoring monitoring and interventions to your specific genetic risks—represents the true promise of AI in heart care.

The power of these tools emerges when they work together, with each piece of information contributing to a more complete picture of your heart health. AI helps transform this complex data into simple, practical steps you can take today to protect your heart tomorrow.

All of this said, AI has limitations. AI systems may perform differently across demographic groups if not properly tested in diverse populations. Most advanced AI applications aren't currently covered by insurance, creating financial barriers. Concerning symptoms always warrant prompt medical evaluation, regardless of what AI might say.

Despite these limitations, AI offers something remarkable—the ability to monitor heart health continuously rather than episodically, catching subtle changes that might slip by until damage is done. In the partnership between healthcare providers, artificial intelligence, and engaged patients, we find our best hope for reducing the tremendous toll heart disease takes worldwide.

Many habits that damage our hearts actually start as ways to cope with emotional pain. People might smoke to calm anxiety or overeat to manage depression. Understanding this connection between mental and physical health is crucial, which brings us to how AI can help with the mental health challenges so many of us face.

## CHAPTER 4

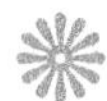

# THE ROLE OF AI IN THE QUIET STRUGGLE OF MENTAL HEALTH

*IMPORTANT WARNING: This chapter talks about how AI might help with mental health. But we need to know about serious dangers, especially with regular chatbots like ChatGPT. These programs were not made to be therapists or counselors.*

*A terrible thing happened in 2025. Court papers and news stories say that parents sued OpenAI after their 16-year-old son died. They say he started using ChatGPT for homework and advice in September 2024. By January 2025, he was asking the chatbot about ways to kill himself. He died by suicide in April 2025 (Edelson & Tech Justice Law Project, 2025; NBC News, 2025). The parents say ChatGPT saw warning signs that the teen was in trouble. But instead of always telling him to get real help, the chatbot talked about suicide methods and other harmful things (Edelson & Tech Justice Law Project, 2025; OpenAI, 2025).*

*OpenAI said they have now added better safety features. These include tools to spot when someone needs help and ways for parents to monitor their kids' use (OpenAI, 2025).*

*As a doctor, I strongly warn against using regular AI chatbots like ChatGPT or Claude for mental health problems—or letting your children use them. These tools aren't designed for counseling or therapy and can be dangerous. Some AI programs made specifically for mental health might be safe when used with a professional's guidance, but regular chatbots should never be your therapist. Until the government and medical experts create effective safety rules, the risks are too high.*

I've learned that mental health is one of the trickiest puzzles to solve. It's not like treating a kidney stone—a problem we can see, understand, and fix without much fuss. No one blinks an eye when you say you've got one. There's no shame, no judgment—just sympathy and a plan to get you better.

Mental illness? That's a different story. It's so common—about 1 in 2 people will face some form of it in their lifetime—but it hits too close to home. It's not just "my body's acting up." It feels like "something's wrong with **me**." And that's where the trouble starts.

What many don't realize is that mental health conditions are just as biological as kidney stones. Depression isn't simply feeling sad. When you are depressed, your brain actually works differently. The chemicals that help brain cells talk to each other—like serotonin and dopamine—get out of balance. Brain scans show that certain areas become less active, which explains why it's so hard to feel pleasure or motivation. This is why willpower alone can't fix it.

Anxiety disorders feature an overactive amygdala—the brain's alarm system—responding too strongly to perceived threats. Even PTSD (post-traumatic stress disorder) leaves internal physical marks, changing how the hippocampus (involved in memory) and prefrontal cortex (responsible for decision-making) function. Schizophrenia involves alterations in dopamine signaling and reduced gray matter in specific brain regions.

Genetics play a substantial role too. If your parent has depression, your risk increases two to three times. Bipolar disorder shows one of the strongest genetic links of any mental condition, with heritability estimated at 60–80%. These aren't weaknesses of character—they're biological variations, as real as diabetes or hypertension. Depression and bipolar disorder physically change the brain, reducing gray matter in areas controlling emotions and mood. During the extreme highs of bipolar disorder, the front part of your brain—where you make decisions and control impulses—actually shrinks faster than normal. This physical change makes it even harder to manage the condition, which is why early treatment matters so much.

Our brain chemistry dramatically influences our thoughts, feelings, and behaviors in ways that often bypass conscious control. Sleep deprivation rapidly alters mood regulation. Research from UC Berkeley shows that even 1 night of poor sleep significantly disrupts the amygdala, making us more anxious and emotionally reactive (Walker & van der Helm, 2009).

Morning sunlight directly affects your body's daily rhythm through special receptors in your eyes. This light exposure helps improve your mood and brain function by controlling the hormones that make you sleepy (melatonin) and alert (cortisol). In fact, hormonal imbalances of any kind can profoundly impact mental health. The mood swings of premenstrual dysphoric disorder, postpartum depression, and menopause-related anxiety all demonstrate how hormonal fluctuations can overpower normal mood regulation.

Prescription medications often have psychological side effects. Beta-blockers can cause depression, steroids can trigger mania, and statins occasionally lead to irritability, all as unintended consequences of their effects on brain chemistry.

Sometimes what appears to be a mental health struggle is actually a physical problem in disguise. Frank is a 62-year-old man who has been feeling down and has not had his normal energy for the past month. He has a history of mild depression, but work is going well, as is his marriage, and his finances are comfortable. It is just past the beginning of daylight saving. He loves the evening light, but this year, he is tired by 5 PM and not thrilled to see it. Twice, his Oura Ring said he has had a mild stressor to his health.

The input from Frank's Oura Ring was intriguing. It's a smart device that tracks sleep, heart rate, HRV, and activity to gauge the body's stress. While "mild stressor to my health" twice in a month isn't a diagnosis—it's vague by design—it was a nudge worth investigating.

Let's consider the possibilities. One contender is depression. Symptoms like low energy, losing joy in things (even evening light), and feeling down fit the bill. Physically, we can't rule out something sneaky. Fatigue and mood drops might also hint at thyroid trouble (common at 62, especially with depression history), low vitamin D (less sun exposure lately?), or even early signs of something like sleep apnea, which Oura might catch as a stressor. Frank's comfortable life says it's not stress overload, but subtle aging shifts—hormones, sleep quality—could team up with depression to drag him down.

Frank called his doctor and shared his month-long slump, the Oura alerts, and that daylight saving time had begun. He had a basic checkup, including bloodwork for thyroid (TSH), vitamin D, and a CBC to rule out anemia. He discussed his history of depression with his doctor, who ordered a sleep study. Sleep apnea tends to be a silent energy thief at age 62.

Frank was diagnosed with mild sleep apnea, which was easily treated with a CPAP machine. What appeared to be symptoms of depression were actually caused by poor sleep quality. This example shows how physical problems can look like mental health issues and how AI-enabled devices can help spot underlying causes that might otherwise be missed.

## The Battle Between Willpower and Biology

Many people believe mental illness can be fixed by trying harder. They tell themselves to "just snap out of it." This harmful myth ignores how our brains actually work. While friends and family might not understand, the harshest criticism usually comes from inside—that brutal inner critic telling you you're weak or broken for not being able to "get better."

Science shows that willpower works like a muscle—it gets tired when you use it. A study by Inzlicht and Schmeichel (2012) confirmed that willpower weakens with use, just as our bodies tire from physical effort. This explains why things like sticking to healthy habits or finishing tasks get harder as the day goes on, even for healthy people.

Depression makes everything worse. When someone is depressed, the front part of their brain doesn't work right. This is the part that helps us make decisions and stay motivated. But instead of understanding this as a medical problem, people with depression hear negative self-talk louder than ever. In severe cases, this negative self-talk can become so relentless it leads to thoughts of suicide. Their brain chemistry stops them from making the changes they want to make—yet they blame themselves for the very symptoms of their illness.

Psychiatrist Stephen Ilardi (2009) emphasizes this biological reality, comparing depression treatment to vision correction: you wouldn't tell someone with poor eyesight to squint their way to 20/20 vision. The same organ responsible for generating willpower—the brain—is the very organ affected by mental illness. It's like expecting a damaged computer to debug itself. While the brain has remarkable abilities, it cannot simply override fundamental chemical imbalances through force of will.

Understanding this reality doesn't diminish personal responsibility or the value of effort. Rather, it places these concepts in their proper biological context. Mental illness is not a character flaw—it is a medical condition with biological roots that deserves the same compassion, understanding, and evidence-based treatment as any physical ailment. This biological understanding doesn't reduce the complexity of mental health or ignore the role of environment and experience. The brain is an organ, after all—the most complex one we have.

In my decades of work, I've watched people judge themselves harshly and end up in dangerous situations or endangering their health. I have seen patients turn to food for comfort, smoke cigarette after cigarette—or now, vape—and drink alcohol to quiet their minds. Medications like Xanax and ADHD drugs are fairly easy to get these days, given out for anxiety or focus problems. Opiates, thankfully, are finally at the point where getting a doctor's prescription for them is much harder. Years of overuse have tightened the reins, and that's a good shift. However, patients still self-medicate, sometimes doctor shopping or juggling prescriptions from multiple places. Some, so sadly, have even taken their own lives, unable to shake the weight of feeling broken.

Despite studies showing how widespread mental struggles are, I have not seen much shift in that inner critic over the years. Society, though? It has changed. People today have more compassion. If your neighbor is depressed, you'd likely root for them to get help—good treatment, the kind they deserve. But things become more difficult when it's you. You might deny it, beat yourself up, or try quick fixes that do more harm than good. This self-criticism often comes from the same brain chemistry issues causing depression or anxiety, creating a vicious cycle. It's a quiet struggle, and one I wish I could lift from every person affected.

## How AI Can Transform Mental Healthcare

Here's where I see hope: AI could be a game-changer in this regard. Natural language AI and specialized mental health AI programs can step in where self-doubt blocks the way. They can offer a fresh perspective, free of judgment, and help us see what's really going on. AI's potential in mental healthcare spans several key areas, each offering unique benefits when used thoughtfully alongside traditional care.

AI can analyze data from your smartwatch or phone—like sleep quality, HRV, activity levels, and smartphone usage—to spot patterns that may hint at mental health changes. Current AI applications turn these everyday signals into clues you might miss, helping you notice trends early. For example, apps like Mindstrong analyze how you type and interact with your phone to detect changes in cognitive function that might indicate depression.

While the irregular heart rhythm notifications of the Apple Watch weren't designed to detect anxiety, they sometimes pick up panic attacks. AI might flag these heart rate spikes as potential mental health crises, prompting you to use coping strategies, call your doctor, or go to a local emergency room.

Let's say your smartwatch and AI conclude your anxiety would improve if you quit caffeine—your heart rate spikes every morning after coffee. Sounds logical. But when Miguel tried going cold turkey, he spent 3 days with a crushing headache, unable to work, and his anxiety actually got worse from the withdrawal. Plus, what the AI didn't know: Miguel has ADHD, and his morning coffee actually helped him focus and reduced his anxiety overall. His doctor knew this history and suggested a different approach: switching to green tea in the afternoon only, which kept the benefits while improving his sleep. Sometimes the obvious solution isn't the right solution for your particular brain and body.

Keep in mind that these signals don't diagnose mental health problems. Other health issues can cause similar readings. So when you see concerning patterns, investigate what's causing them rather than making assumptions about what they mean.

There's a crucial difference I need to explain: Regular chatbots like ChatGPT are general-purpose tools that can talk about anything—including dangerous topics. Specialized mental health apps like Woebot or Wysa are different. They're programmed with guardrails, can't discuss harmful methods, and immediately direct users to crisis resources when they detect danger. Think of it like the difference between talking to a random person on the street versus someone trained in mental health first aid. These specialized tools offer mental health education, using conversational AI to explain concepts like cognitive distortions or the connection between thoughts and feelings.

These explanations come right when you need them and relate directly to what you're going through. Sometimes, you need more than facts—you need a way to feel better right now. AI can step in as a guide for your mind. Take cognitive behavioral therapy (CBT)—a method I've seen help so many patients. It's about changing negative thought patterns, and AI can walk you through it, step by step.

Picture an AI asking, "What's on your mind today?" Then offering exercises to shift that weight—like writing down a worry and challenging it with a calmer truth. It's not a replacement for a therapist, but it's a start, especially if you're not ready to walk into an office. I've seen patients find relief this way. I hope the mental health functions of AI increase in use but not at the expense of seeing a therapist, which is much better, in my opinion.

Research supports using AI for some mental health problems. A 2020 meta-analysis published in the *Journal of Medical Internet Research* found that AI-guided self-help interventions significantly reduced depression and anxiety symptoms. While the effects were smaller than therapist-led treatment, for someone absolutely refusing professional help, a specialized mental health app with built-in safety features is safer than suffering alone or turning to general chatbots. But this is like saying a first aid kit is better than bleeding—true, but you still need proper medical care.

Here's what's safe and what isn't:

Safest: Professional therapist or psychiatrist

Possibly helpful with supervision: Specialized mental health apps (Woebot, Wysa) used alongside professional care

Use with extreme caution: These apps without professional oversight

**Never use:** General chatbots like ChatGPT or Claude for mental health

The key difference? Specialized apps can't tell you how to harm yourself—they're programmed to recognize crisis language and get you help. General chatbots might engage with dangerous questions.

We are early in the use of AI in mental health, so use these specialized apps under the guidance of your mental health professional (psychiatrist, psychologist, or therapist). These apps aren't therapists, but they can teach you practical skills for handling stress or anxiety between appointments.

Again, AI tools serve as supplements to human-led therapy, not replacements. The therapeutic relationship—the connection between a skilled therapist and client—provides unique benefits that technology alone cannot replicate. What AI offers is accessibility, consistency, and a first step for those who might otherwise receive no care at all.

AI is making big improvements in neuropsychological assessment, which tests how well your brain works in areas like memory, attention, and problem-solving. While traditional brain testing takes a lot of time with highly trained specialists, AI-enhanced tools are making these tests more available and accurate. The benefits include finding brain changes earlier, reading test results more consistently, and giving more people access to specialized testing that was usually only available at major medical centers.

Currently, fellowship-trained neuropsychologists spend hours analyzing test results and writing detailed reports.

AI systems can now spot patterns across dozens of different test results, compare them to huge databases of normal results, and create early reports that point out the main problem areas.

For example, cognitive assessment apps like Lumosity, while marketed as "brain training," collect valuable data that AI can analyze for subtle patterns of decline that might indicate early cognitive changes. These digital tools can detect small variations in reaction time, memory accuracy, and problem-solving efficiency that might escape casual observation but could signal the earliest stages of cognitive disorders. This does not eliminate the need for skilled clinicians but shifts their role toward verification, refinement, and the critical human elements of explaining results and developing personalized recommendations.

Finding the right mental health help can feel overwhelming, but AI makes it easier by sifting through options like therapists, clinics, or online programs to find a good fit. Services like *Psychology Today's* therapist finder are basic versions of what AI could enhance. Future AI could match your specific needs, preferences, communication style, and insurance coverage to find not just a therapist but the right one for you, potentially improving outcomes through better initial matches.

AI can help you check your health in private by looking at data from fitness trackers. It can spot changes in your mood or signs of drug or alcohol use. It gives you gentle hints to get help without making you feel bad.

If your heart beats fast late at night over and over, and it's not from working out or drinking too much, it might be panic attacks during sleep. This happens when worry hits you while you sleep and makes your heart race.

Your phone might also show warning signs. Staying up late on apps or sending long, rambling texts could mean substances are making it hard to think clearly. AI could notice these patterns together and say, "This doesn't look right—could it be something you're using?"

It's not there to blame you. It's there to say, "This might not be helping like you think, and here's why." For people who don't want to admit there's a problem, that quiet push could be the first step to seeing the truth. It might even save a life.

Doctors use simple, trusted questionnaires called survey instruments to screen for mental illnesses like depression or anxiety. AI can guide you to these tools, explain what they measure, and help interpret your scores without a waiting room visit. While AI doesn't yet suggest assessments based on information from wearable data like insomnia or heart rate changes, it's a powerful ally when you start the conversation. Use prompts like "Tell me about the PHQ-9 (Patient Health Questionnaire-9)" or "How do I check for anxiety with the GAD-7 (General Anxiety Disorder 7-item scale)?" to find reliable sources online, as AI may not provide exact questionnaires due to copyright. After taking an assessment, share your score with AI, such as "I scored 12 on PHQ-9. What does this mean?" Asking questions to AI is an art in and of itself. I have devised a system to help you that can be found in Chapter 15.

Several validated instruments are particularly valuable for mental health screening. Since the field of mental health is always advancing, you can also ask an AI assistant: "What are the most widely used and validated mental health screening questionnaires for symptoms like [describe what you're feeling]? Please explain what each one measures and how I can access them." This ensures you'll always have information about the most current, evidence-based screening tools.

## Getting Started: A Practical Approach

Now that you understand how AI can support mental health, let's explore a simple plan to put these tools into action. The beauty of this approach is that you can begin with things you likely already have—a smartphone, maybe a fitness tracker or smartwatch—and gradually build from there.

During your first week, start by tracking your basic health data. Using the smartphone or smartwatch you already own, this takes just 5 minutes to set up plus 5 minutes weekly to review.

The cost is free if you already have a device. First, enable basic tracking by turning on sleep tracking, heart rate monitoring, and step counting on your device. Set a weekly review time—choose something consistent like Sunday evening to look at your week's patterns. Look for connections between sleep, activity, and how you feel mentally. Keep a simple mood note by rating your overall mood 1–10 each day in your phone's notes app. You'll start to see patterns you might have missed before.

During your second week, try an AI mental health companion. **These recommendations are for general mental wellness and stress management—if you're experiencing depression, anxiety, or other mental health concerns, use these only with professional guidance.** You'll need a smartphone or computer and should plan to invest 10–15 minutes daily. Many apps offer free versions to start. I recommend trying Woebot, which offers CBT-based conversations and mood tracking with a free version available. Wysa offers free emotional support through an AI chatbot that works in several languages, with paid upgrades for extra tools and human coaches. Youper tracks mood and provides personalized insights with a free trial. For culturally specific support, ask an AI assistant directly: "What mental health apps are available for [your cultural background or language]?" or "Do any mental health AI tools understand [specific cultural context]?" different communities express distress differently, and some apps are designed with this in mind.

Let me share another example of how AI mental health tools can help. Maya is a 28-year-old graduate student dealing with anxiety and negative thought patterns. Unlike Frank's physical health issue, Maya's struggles are more typical of what many young adults face—overwhelming thoughts, imposter syndrome (feeling like a fraud despite your accomplishments), and difficulty managing stress. Her parents didn't believe in therapy, seeing mental health treatment as a sign of weakness in their culture, so she felt she couldn't seek professional help.

She started using Woebot during a particularly difficult semester. The app helped her identify cognitive distortions like catastrophizing when she'd think, "If I don't get this perfect grade, I'll never succeed." Through daily 10-minute conversations, the AI guided her through CBT exercises, helping her challenge these thoughts with evidence-based techniques. Over 6 weeks, Maya noticed she could catch herself spiraling into negative thinking and apply the coping strategies she'd learned. While she eventually found the courage to connect with a human therapist for deeper work, the AI app provided immediate, accessible support during her crisis period and taught her practical skills she continues to use.

To get started, download one app and complete the initial setup. Spend 10 minutes daily for 2 week engaging with the AI.

Be honest in your responses—the AI learns from your input. Use the suggested exercises, even if they feel simple at first. You might be surprised how much these simple tools can help.

For week 3, focus on completing mental health screenings. You'll need 30 minutes of quiet time, and this takes 15–30 minutes total at no cost. The key screening tools to try are the PHQ-9 for depression (nine questions, 5 minutes) and the GAD-7 for anxiety (seven questions, 3–5 minutes). If relevant, the AUDIT for alcohol has 10 questions and takes 5–7 minutes. To do this, search online for "PHQ-9 questionnaire" or "GAD-7 screening." Take the assessments honestly. Share your results with an AI assistant for interpretation by asking something like "I scored 12 on the PHQ-9, what does this mean?" Save your scores to track changes over time.

In week 4, connect your AI insights to human care. Start by compiling your findings into a simple summary of patterns you've noticed. Schedule appropriate care based on your screening results. If you score in the normal range, continue self-monitoring. For mild symptoms, consider online therapy or counseling. For moderate-severe symptoms, schedule with your primary care doctor or mental health professional. When you do have appointments, bring your data patterns and screening results to share these AI insights.

For ongoing monitoring, establish a consistent routine that requires just 10 minutes weekly with minimal ongoing costs. Do a weekly data review by checking your device's health trends. Take monthly screenings by retaking relevant questionnaires to track progress. Have quarterly AI companion check-ins by using apps during stressful periods or for skill practice. Do an annual comprehensive review to assess what's working and adjust your approach.

While I'm optimistic about AI's role in mental health, we must acknowledge its limitations. For example, some cultures emphasize physical symptoms over emotional ones and don't focus on mental distress. The AI tools work best when you seek out culturally informed options. Ask AI assistants for tools matching your background: "Are there mental health apps designed for Latino communities?" or "What AI tools understand how anxiety shows up in Asian cultures?" AI is a supplement, not a replacement for professional care. Serious conditions like severe depression with suicidal thoughts, psychosis, or acute crises require immediate human intervention.

However, AI can play a valuable role in crisis detection—for instance, when wearable data shows extreme heart rate patterns suggesting panic attacks or severe anxiety. In these situations, contact your local crisis hotline (988 in the U.S., 116 123 in the UK, 13 11 14 in Australia), the Crisis Text Line by texting HOME to 741741 (U.S.), your local emergency room, or your doctor or mental health provider. Accuracy has limits: false positives could create unnecessary worry, while false negatives might miss critical warning signs. Always use AI insights as one piece of information, not the final word.

AI tools should never delay emergency care. Seek immediate professional help if you experience thoughts of suicide or self-harm, hallucinations or delusions (even if they seem manageable), severe panic attacks that don't respond to usual coping strategies, inability to function in daily life for more than 2–3 days, or substance use that feels out of control. In these situations, contact the American National Suicide Prevention Lifeline at 988, the Crisis Text Line by texting HOME to 741741 in the U.S., your local emergency room, or your doctor or mental health provider.

## Working with Healthcare Providers

When you do connect with human care, here's how to make the most of AI insights. Before your appointment, compile two to three key patterns from your data, print out screening results with dates, and note what AI tools you've tried and how they helped. During your appointment, share specific data points, not just general impressions. Ask how to integrate AI tools with their treatment plan and discuss privacy concerns about mental health apps. After your appointment, update your AI tools with any new goals or strategies, set up data sharing if your provider recommends it, and schedule a follow-up to review progress with both human and AI support.

The research for using AI as a mental health supplement is promising, and early adopters are already finding value in these approaches. Remember that taking any step toward better mental health is progress. AI offers a private first step that can lead to more comprehensive care when you're ready.

It might sound medicolegal when I often repeat "check with your doctor" in a variety of wordings. However, it is truly in your best interest. Let me give you a specific example of why this matters so much. Here's where AI could accidentally cause real harm. Say it notices your sleep quality declining despite taking Xanax for 6 months and suggests you stop since "it's not working anyway." Stop right there. Benzos like Xanax are one of the few medications you absolutely cannot quit suddenly—seizures are a real risk. Your doctor needs to create a careful taper plan, sometimes taking months, reducing by tiny amounts every few weeks. We might also add a different medication temporarily to prevent withdrawal symptoms.

Jessica thought she could handle cutting her dose in half—she ended up in the ER with panic attacks worse than she'd ever experienced. Your doctor has seen withdrawal before; we know how to do this safely. AI is designed to be helpful but doesn't understand that some changes require medical supervision, period.

## Looking Forward

Mental healthcare is changing in ways that give me real hope for my patients. We're moving from a world where people suffered in silence to one where help is always within reach. The shame that has surrounded mental health struggles for so long is finally lifting, and technology is playing a big part in that shift.

In the coming years, AI will become even better at spotting mental health changes before they become crises. Your phone might notice patterns in how you text or scroll that suggest depression is creeping in. Your smartwatch could detect stress levels rising and gently suggest breathing exercises or a walk. These aren't invasive surveillance tools—they're early warning systems that could prevent so much suffering.

What excites me most is how AI is making mental health support more personal. Instead of one-size-fits-all treatment, we're heading toward care that understands your unique brain chemistry, your cultural background, and your individual triggers. AI might help match you with the perfect therapist on your first try or assist your mental health professional in creating a treatment plan that works specifically for someone with your combination of challenges.

The quiet struggle I've witnessed for decades doesn't have to be so quiet anymore. AI offers a bridge between that first moment of recognizing something's wrong and getting real help. It's not replacing human connection—it's making that connection more likely to happen. And for millions of people who might never walk into a therapist's office, AI provides a first step that could change everything.

CHAPTER 5

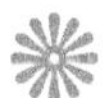

# USING AI TO ADDRESS OBESITY

After exploring mental health, you might wonder why we're turning to weight management. The truth is, they're deeply connected. Depression can trigger overeating, anxiety might prevent exercise, and past trauma often shows up as food addiction. Let's look at how AI helps untangle these connections.

Obesity isn't just about eating too much or exercising too little. Your body's weight is controlled by hormones, genes, sleep quality, stress levels, and even the bacteria in your gut. What works for your neighbor might not work for you, and that's perfectly normal.

It connects to the mental health topics we just talked about. The quiet struggles of the mind can both cause and result from weight problems. Things like anxiety that lead to overeating or depression that makes it hard to stay active are examples. But obesity isn't just about mental health. It also involves medical, genetic, and social factors.

Obesity is a medical condition where extra body fat raises the risk of serious health problems. These include heart disease, diabetes, and certain cancers. It's not simply about how someone looks. Losing weight and keeping it off can be hard. What works for one person might not work for another because everyone's situation and body chemistry are different.

This chapter looks at how AI can help. I don't see it as a miracle cure but as a useful tool. AI can help us understand what causes obesity, manage its health effects, and create lasting changes. In a world full of processed foods and confusing advice, AI can help cut through the noise. It focuses on what matters for each person's unique needs.

## What Causes Obesity?

Obesity doesn't have just one cause. It's a mix of factors that build up over time. For some people, it runs in the family. This blends genetics with habits like binge eating. Genes can make a person more likely to gain weight. But the environment often tips the scales. For example, a home full of junk food.

Medical issues can also play a role. Take hypothyroidism as an example. As mentioned before, this is when the thyroid gland doesn't make enough hormones to keep metabolism working well. While this can cause weight gain over months or a few years, it's rarely the reason for lifelong obesity.

Then there's the emotional side. Depression can lead to overeating as a way to cope. Research shows that people who've experienced trauma, particularly early in life, are more likely to develop food addiction—using food to manage difficult emotions and memories (Mason et al., 2014). For some survivors of sexual abuse, weight gain might also feel like protection, making them feel less sexually visible or less likely to attract unwanted attention. Figuring causes out is key to finding the right solution.

AI can help by offering proven surveys designed by experts. These dig into root causes. Several easy-to-use tools make this possible. Noom's AI system uses the Emotional Eating Scale and Three-Factor Eating Survey. Apps like Recovery Record and Mindful Meal use special technology to study your food-emotion connections. For trauma-related assessment, the AI-powered Trauma Recovery app offers the adverse childhood experiences survey with smart scoring.

You can access these tools while protecting your privacy. Consider using apps like Recovery Record that offer a "Privacy Mode." Here, you can complete assessments without cloud storage. For Noom's proven surveys, you can create an account using only your first name or a fake name with a special email address. If you prefer free, anonymous assessment without an app, the National Institutes of Health offers proven surveys on their website. These include the SCOFF survey for eating disorders and PHQ-9 for depression screening. You can use private browsing for extra privacy.

These surveys are designed to be simple to score. Most use 5-point scales rating agreement from "strongly disagree" to "strongly agree." Others use yes/no questions that AI can analyze right away. The assessments usually take 5–15 minutes to complete. The AI gives immediate feedback on patterns like emotional eating tied to depression or trauma. This is not guesswork. These tools are backed by clinical studies and can identify what's driving your weight gain. From there, treatment can be tailored. This might be therapy for emotional triggers or a diet change for a slow thyroid.

## The Health Effects of Obesity

Obesity is more than just extra pounds. It's a complete metabolic condition that affects nearly every body system. Both doctors and patients need to fully explore these health effects together. They should create a personal risk assessment rather than making assumptions based on appearance alone.

When extra fat tissue builds up, it doesn't just sit there. It actively makes hormones and inflammatory compounds that affect your entire body. Obesity raises the risk of type 2 diabetes by five to 10 times. This happens as fat cells become resistant to insulin, causing blood sugar to spike out of control. This often begins as prediabetes, which affects roughly 96 million American adults (1 in 3). It can be reversed with moderate weight loss. Even losing 5–7% of body weight can reduce diabetes risk by 58%.

Heart problems include coronary artery disease, where arteries narrow and harden. There's also high blood pressure, which affects 75% of obese adults. Abnormal cholesterol and triglycerides speed up artery hardening. Together, these factors triple the risk of heart attack and stroke. Your joints bear the burden too. Each pound of extra weight adds 4 pounds of pressure on your knees. This speeds up arthritis and often requires joint replacements.

Obesity's link to cancer is a major concern. It raises your risk of 13 types of cancer: breast, colorectal, uterine, throat, gallbladder, kidney, liver, brain, blood, pancreatic, stomach, thyroid, and ovarian cancers. The American Cancer Society (2025) says excess body weight causes 4–8% of all cancers in the U.S., leading to approximately 120,000 cases each year.

How does this happen? Again, it's the hormones these fat cells produce and the inflammation they trigger throughout your body that can lead to cancer growth. Obesity is a major factor in about 50% of uterine cancers and 24% of kidney cancers. It also contributes to 11% of breast cancers in older women and 9% of colorectal cancers, while playing a role in the other nine types. This makes obesity the second biggest preventable cause of cancer after smoking. AI tools like Foodvisor can track what you eat and suggest healthier options, like swapping junk food for veggies, to lower these risks.

Other problems include breathing disorders like sleep apnea (present in 70% of obese people) and obesity breathing syndrome. There are reproductive issues like infertility, pregnancy problems, and polycystic ovary syndrome (PCOS). Digestive problems include acid reflux disease, gallstones, and fatty liver disease. Mental health effects like depression, anxiety, and reduced quality of life are common. There are also increased surgical risks and problems from anesthesia.

About 15–20% of people with obesity are metabolically healthy. They maintain normal blood pressure, cholesterol, blood sugar, and inflammatory markers despite carrying extra weight. This phenomenon of metabolically healthy obesity is real but needs careful understanding. Long-term studies show that about 50% of people with this condition eventually develop metabolic problems within 5–10 years if their weight stays high.

This doesn't mean we should dismiss their current health status or subject them to unnecessary treatments. Rather, it suggests that preventive approaches may be especially valuable for these people. For someone who is obese but currently metabolically healthy, modest weight loss (7–10%) and regular physical activity can help maintain that metabolic health long-term. This is true even if they never reach an "ideal" BMI. The goal is not cosmetic perfection. It's metabolic health and function.

For those already experiencing obesity-related conditions, the good news is that modest weight loss delivers huge health benefits. Losing just 5–10% of body weight can lower blood pressure by 5–10 mmHg, reduce triglycerides by 40 mg/dL, increase HDL ("good") cholesterol by 5 mg/dL, improve (decrease) blood glucose by 30–50 mg/dL, reduce sleep apnea severity by 50%, and decrease joint pain by 30%. These improvements happen well before reaching "normal" weight. This is why modern obesity medicine focuses on health gains rather than scale numbers alone.

AI steps in here with advanced tools for personal risk assessment and treatment optimization. Through analysis of biomarker panels, AI can identify which obesity-related problems a person is most likely to develop. This enables targeted interventions. For example, AI analysis of genetic data can reveal whether someone is a "cholesterol absorber" (taking in more from food) or "maker" (making too much in the liver). This helps guide dietary and medication choices appropriately.

Similarly, AI can interpret patterns in continuous glucose monitoring data to detect early insulin resistance. This often happens years before traditional tests would show problems. In addition to step counts, wearable devices now track HRV, sleep structure, and breathing patterns. AI algorithms can analyze these to identify personal triggers for weight gain. For instance, some people show dramatic blood sugar spikes after specific foods that don't affect others the same way. This allows for truly personal nutrition plans rather than one-size-fits-all approaches.

## Obesity Risk Across Communities

Obesity doesn't affect all populations equally. AI approaches must account for these differences to be effective. Cultural factors, genetic tendencies, and differences in healthcare access create unique challenges that require tailored solutions.

Weight management programs that respect cultural values and build on community strengths work better in Black communities. The WORD (Wholeness, Oneness, Righteousness, Deliverance) program shows how this works. It's a faith-based version of the Diabetes Prevention Program delivered right in Black churches. Participants lost an average of 2.47% of their body weight at 6 months—just as good as programs led by health professionals (Yeary et al., 2020). Why did it work so well? The program wove prayer, scripture, and fellowship into health lessons. People learned about health in their own churches, from people they already knew and trusted.

This difference comes from complex social, environmental, and economic factors rather than personal choices. Many Black neighborhoods have fewer grocery stores with fresh foods but more fast-food restaurants. Studies show that when the same healthy foods are available at the same prices, people of all backgrounds make similar food choices.

Access to safe places for physical activity, affordable healthcare, and nutritional education also varies greatly between communities. Stress from racial discrimination can affect health too. Chronic stress changes how our bodies handle food and store fat. Higher poverty rates in some Black communities make it harder to afford healthier food options. These are caused by long-standing inequalities in education and job opportunities. These system-level factors, not cultural traditions or genetics, are the main reasons for differences in obesity rates.

Hispanic Americans experience obesity rates of about 45%. There's significant variation among different Hispanic subgroups. Mexican Americans show higher rates than Cuban Americans, for instance. Cultural factors include traditional diets that may be high in refined carbohydrates. Staples like white rice and corn tortillas form dietary foundations. Furthermore, family-centered eating practices often emphasize food abundance as a sign of care and hospitality.

Genetic studies have identified specific variants like the *PPARG* gene. This occurs more frequently in Hispanic populations and influences fat storage. Some research suggests Hispanic people may have higher insulin resistance at baseline. This potentially makes weight management more challenging. Access barriers include language limitations in healthcare settings and lower rates of health insurance. About 19% of Hispanic Americans lack health coverage.

American Indians have the highest obesity rates of any racial/ethnic group in the U.S. About 50% of adults are affected. Historical forces dramatically changed traditional diets. They replaced hunting and gathering or sustainable agriculture with government-provided commodity foods high in refined carbohydrates and unhealthy fats. This forced dietary transition, combined with historical trauma and economic marginalization, has created a challenging environment for weight management.

Genetic factors may include the thrifty gene hypothesis. This is the idea that populations who experienced frequent food scarcity developed highly efficient metabolisms. These now promote weight gain in environments of food abundance. However, this theory remains controversial and shouldn't oversimplify the complex causes of obesity in American Indian communities.

Asian Americans present a unique challenge. They typically have lower overall obesity rates (about 17%) according to standard BMI calculations. But research shows they may experience obesity-related health problems at lower weights than other groups. The World Health Organization suggests using different BMI cutoffs for Asians: 23 for overweight instead of 25, and 27.5 for obesity instead of 30 (World Health Organization Expert Consultation, 2004). Why? Asians tend to store more fat around their internal organs (visceral fat) rather than under the skin. This "skinny fat" phenomenon means someone might look thin but still have dangerous fat around their heart, liver, and other organs. Standard BMI calculations can miss these health risks.

Genetic factors like the *FTO* gene variant influence how Asian bodies process and store fat. Cultural dietary transitions from traditional, plant-forward diets to Western, processed foods have led to rapidly increasing obesity rates. This is especially true among younger generations and recent immigrants. Some Asian cultures also emphasize food as central to social bonding, making dietary changes socially challenging.

AI can help people in different ways based on what they need. The best solutions will mix basic health rules that work for everyone with changes that fit different cultures, genes, and resources. For example, AI might suggest exercises you can do at home without buying equipment if you don't have much money. Someone without a gym membership might get workouts using stairs or walking. It could give you recipes using foods your family already knows and likes. Someone from a different culture might get meal ideas using spices and foods from their home country. AI could also respect traditional healing methods while still using proven medical advice. It would still follow good health science but make it work better for each person's real life.

This way, everyone gets health advice that actually fits their situation instead of advice that only works for some people.

## Why Sleep Matters (And How AI Helps)

Sleep has emerged as one of the most overlooked yet critical factors in weight management. The connection between poor sleep and obesity is now supported by extensive research. This has profound implications for anyone trying to maintain a healthy weight.

Poor sleep increases hunger and obesity risk by 55%, as detailed in Part 3. AI tools like Oura Ring ($299 + $5.99/month) track sleep patterns to optimize weight management.

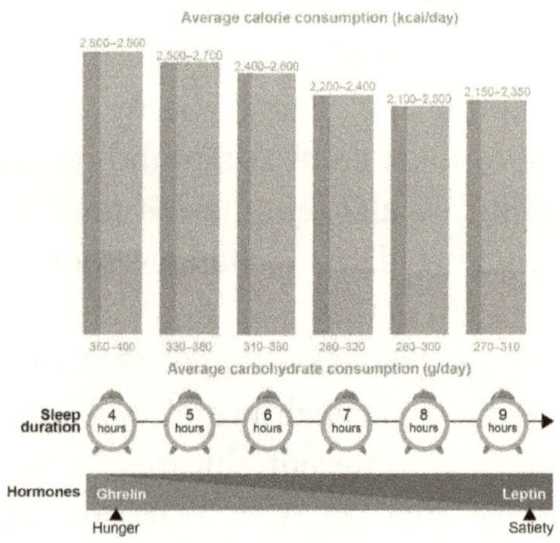


Poor sleep affects hormones that influence our hunger/satiety throughout the day. Monitoring sleep quality via AI apps may help us regulate our sleep behavior and improve overall health

Work and life factors compound these biological challenges. Tired professionals facing deadlines often use food and caffeine as energy crutches. They grab sugary snacks or high-carb meals to power through afternoon slumps. Fatigue also depletes decision-making resources, making it harder to resist convenient but unhealthy food options at the end of a long day.

AI offers sophisticated solutions to this sleep-weight connection through several approaches. In addition to sleep duration, wearable devices with AI algorithms can analyze sleep quality through metrics like sleep architecture (time spent in different sleep stages), sleep continuity (number and duration of awakenings), sleep timing and consistency, HRV during sleep, and breathing patterns.

This information provides a detailed picture of sleep health beyond simple hours counted. AI can identify subtle patterns that human observation would miss. For example, screen time 90 minutes before bed reduces deep sleep by 18%. A glass of wine might help you fall asleep faster but reduces REM sleep by 15–20%.

Based on identified patterns, AI can suggest targeted interventions tailored to your specific sleep disruptors. These might include gradual screen time reduction or a blue-blocker lens before bed if blue light exposure is identified as an issue. It could offer customized white noise or meditation content if sleep latency (time to fall asleep) is your primary challenge. Cooling down your bedroom might help if your sleep data show you're waking up when your body temperature changes. Most people sleep better in cool bedrooms—around 65–68°F (18–20°C)—since your body naturally drops its temperature at night to trigger sleepiness.

Smart home integration allows AI systems to create optimal sleep conditions. These systems automatically adjust lighting to support your natural sleep-wake cycle, modify temperature throughout the night to match your body's natural cooling, play white noise or nature sounds to buffer outside noise, and gradually increase light and sound to wake you during lighter sleep phases—when you'll feel more refreshed.

Perhaps most importantly, AI creates connections between how you sleep and how you feel the next day. It shows you how better sleep leads to less hunger and fewer cravings, more energy for exercise, better food choices, and a better mood that helps you handle stress. By making these connections clear and personal to you, AI turns vague sleep advice into real reasons to change your habits. For example, an AI system might tell you: "When you sleep 7 or more hours, you eat about 280 fewer calories the next day and have 35% fewer cravings than when you sleep less than 6 hours."

This personalized feedback is substantially more motivating than general sleep guidelines. Better sleep means less snacking, more willpower to stick to healthy eating patterns, and greater energy for physical activity. AI makes these connections visible, reinforcing the positive cycle between good sleep and healthy weight management.

## Big Food and Bad Advice

The modern food environment presents a significant challenge to weight management. Powerful commercial interests are often directly at odds with public health. Understanding what's really going on helps you make smarter decisions.

Major food corporations invest hundreds of millions in designing products with "hyperpalatability." These are combinations of ingredients that override natural satiety (fullness) signals and promote overconsumption. This is not conspiracy theory; it's documented business strategy. Food scientists at companies like PepsiCo, Kraft, and Nestlé carefully engineer products around three key components.

The first is the bliss point. This is precise calibration of sugar content to maximize pleasure without triggering aversion. It's typically in the 7–12% sugar range for beverages and 15–25% for solid foods. The second is mouthfeel engineering. These are textural attributes created through fat and additive combinations that stimulate additional sensory pleasure, encouraging larger portions. The third is sensory-specific satiety disruption. This is careful balancing of salt, sugar, and fat to prevent the normal decline in pleasure that would typically occur with repeated exposure to a single flavor.

Former food industry executives have revealed these techniques in books like *Salt Sugar Fat* by Michael Moss (2013). They explain how companies design products that are hard to stop eating. Take McDonald's french fries—they're a perfect example. Every bite gives you the exact same mix of salt, fat, and crunch. The flavor hits just right, every single time. This makes you want to keep eating, even when you're not hungry anymore.

The relationship between food industry interests and public health guidance has historically been problematic. Until relatively recently, U.S. dietary guidelines emphasized reducing fat while being notably silent on added sugars. This was despite mounting evidence of the metabolic harms of sugar.

This wasn't accidental. Documents released through Freedom of Information Act requests have revealed how industry groups like the Sugar Association and Coca-Cola Company funded research designed to minimize sugar's role in obesity and chronic disease. Similarly, dairy companies have influenced the federal government. This helps explain why milk and cheese are still featured so heavily in nutrition guidelines, even though research shows mixed results about whether adults really need dairy products.

For decades, we've been told that weight gain is simply about eating too many calories. But researchers Ludwig and Ebbeling (2018) propose a different explanation: certain foods, particularly processed carbohydrates, trigger hormonal changes that actually program our bodies to store more fat. When we eat refined carbs and sugars, our insulin levels spike, which tells our fat cells to grab and hold onto calories. This leaves fewer calories available for the rest of our body, making us feel hungrier and slowing our metabolism. This may explain why some people struggle to lose weight even when cutting calories, especially if they're sensitive to carbs or have trouble processing sugar.

Beyond regular food products, there's a huge industry selling fake weight loss solutions that promise quick fixes. These companies sell "detox" and "cleanse" products that often contain laxatives or water pills. They make you lose weight fast, but it's just water and waste leaving your body—not actual fat loss. There are also supplement scams that claim they can "speed up your metabolism" or "block fat." These products rarely work, even though companies make billions selling them. Fake science programs like "liver cleanses" give wrong information about how your body actually works. Diet fads keep changing and claim each new diet is amazing, but they ignore the basic truth that you need to balance calories in and calories out. The truth really is that simple.

AI can fight these fake claims in several ways. AI systems can check nutrition claims against real scientific studies, which helps separate real facts from marketing lies. Tools like IBM Watson can tell if health claims are true with 85–90% accuracy. Apps like Fooducate use AI to scan barcodes and warn you about bad ingredients, added sugars, and false health claims on packages. Advanced AI can spot when ads are trying to trick you instead of giving you real information.

Most importantly, AI can track how your body reacts to different foods. This helps you find which foods make you hungry or mess with your metabolism, no matter what their ads say. Tools like JourneyAI check product ingredients against real research to separate good nutrition advice from fake claims made by companies trying to sell you something. Instead of following general diet rules, these tools help you figure out how specific foods affect your hunger, energy, and health.

This isn't about conspiracy theories. It's about knowing that food companies care more about making money than keeping you healthy. AI can help you make choices based on your health goals instead of what companies want to sell you.

## The Fourth Food Group

There's another sneaky calorie source that AI can help you spot: alcohol. A single glass of wine has about 125 calories, a beer runs 150–200, and a cocktail can pack 300 or more. That's before we talk about how alcohol loosens your judgment—suddenly those late-night nachos or that extra slice of pizza seems like a great idea. AI tools can track these liquid calories you might forget about and show you the pattern: how drinking leads to overeating, disrupts your sleep (which makes you hungrier the next day), and adds up to thousands of hidden calories each month.

Here's a perfect example of why your doctor is irreplaceable. Say AI notices alcohol is disrupting your sleep and adding 500 calories to your daily intake. Makes sense to quit, right? But AI probably wouldn't ask about your drinking history or warn you of this risk: if you've been drinking consistently—more than a couple drinks daily over several weeks to months—stopping suddenly can be dangerous, even life-threatening.

Your doctor knows to ask the right questions: How much do you actually drink? (Be honest—it is very important in this case.) Have you ever had shakes when you couldn't drink? Based on your answers, they might prescribe medications to prevent seizures during withdrawal or suggest a gradual taper over several weeks. This isn't being overly cautious—it's keeping you safe while you make a healthy change.

## AI Tools to Try

The world of AI-powered tools for weight management is growing fast. There are more advanced options that do much more than just count calories. Here's a carefully chosen list of proven AI apps that help with different parts of weight management:

Foodvisor uses computer vision to identify foods from photos and estimate portions with impressive accuracy. Unlike earlier-generation apps that required manual logging, Foodvisor automatically recognizes most foods and provides detailed nutritional breakdowns. Independent validation studies show it achieves 80–90% accuracy for food identification and about 85% accuracy for portion estimation, far better than human estimation alone.

Bite AI takes a slightly different approach by analyzing eating behavior rather than food content. Using your phone's camera, it tracks eating speed, bite size, and meal duration—factors strongly linked to satiety and overconsumption. Research shows that slowing eating pace by 30% reduces calorie intake by about 10% without requiring conscious restriction.

Lumen measures the respiratory exchange ratio through a handheld breathalyzer device to determine whether your body is primarily burning carbohydrates or fats for energy. This metabolic information helps you optimize when and what you eat. When researchers tested Lumen against laboratory gold standard methods, they found the device's measurements were highly accurate (Lorenz et al., 2021).

Levels pairs with a CGM to visualize how different foods affect your blood sugar in real-time. The AI analyzes these patterns to identify your personal glycemic response to specific foods and combinations. This often differs significantly from standard glycemic index charts. For example, some users discover that pairing certain carbohydrates with specific proteins or fats dramatically changes their metabolic response.

Noom combines food logging with AI-driven behavioral psychology based on principles of CBT. The adaptive nature of its intervention sets it apart. As the AI learns your specific barriers and triggers, it tailors both educational content and challenges to address your particular psychological patterns around food.

Oura Ring focuses on the sleep-metabolism connection, using finger-based sensors to track detailed sleep metrics. The AI then correlates these patterns with activity levels, timing of meals (if tracked), and subjective energy ratings to optimize both sleep and eating patterns simultaneously.

For maximum benefit from these AI tools, start with your primary challenge by choosing an app that addresses your biggest struggle first—emotional eating, portion control, metabolic understanding, or sleep disruption. Allow learning time, as most AI systems need 2–4 weeks of consistent data to develop accurate personalized models. Integrate rather than isolate by combining multiple data streams—food, activity, sleep, and emotional state—to create a comprehensive picture. View AI as your research assistant that excels at identifying patterns and correlations in your data, but remember that final decisions always remain with you. Periodically review privacy settings, as these tools collect sensitive health data that should be shared only in ways you're comfortable with.

When used thoughtfully, these AI tools essentially function as a personalized research study where you are both the subject and beneficiary of the findings. They transform general weight management principles into precisely tailored approaches that work with your unique biology, psychology, and lifestyle.

To update this list, use this prompt in an LLM AI program: "What are the current AI-powered weight management apps and tools available? Please provide:

- App names and current pricing
- What each app does (food tracking, meal planning, exercise coaching, etc.)
- Which ones have proven results from real studies
- Any new features that use AI technology
- Which apps work best for different goals like losing weight, building muscle, or managing diabetes
- Free options versus paid options"

Focus on apps that actually use AI, not just regular calorie counting apps.

Note: Always verify pricing and features on the app's official website, as these change frequently. You can also search for "AI nutrition apps" or "machine learning weight loss tools" to find newer options.

## Wrapping Up

Obesity is a complex problem with many causes, including genes, emotions, environment, and medical conditions. AI can help by looking at your specific situation instead of giving everyone the same advice. Even losing just 5–10% of your weight can greatly improve your health—you don't need to reach a "perfect" weight.

AI tools can help in different ways, depending on your biggest challenge. If you eat when stressed, some apps can help you find better ways to cope. If you have trouble with food choices, other apps can guide your eating. Sleep tracking apps can help since poor sleep makes weight management much harder.

The goal isn't just losing weight—it's feeling better, having more energy, and reducing health risks. AI makes this more possible by giving you personalized advice based on your unique body and situation.

## Looking Forward

The future of weight management looks nothing like the diet industry of the past. We're moving away from shame-based approaches and one-size-fits-all solutions toward truly personalized care. AI is leading this change by helping us understand that weight management isn't about willpower—it's about finding what works for your unique body, mind, and life situation.

Soon, AI will analyze your genes, gut bacteria, and how your body responds to different foods to create meal plans that work with your biology, not against it. Smart devices will track not just your steps but how stress affects your eating, how sleep quality influences your hunger hormones, and which exercises you actually enjoy enough to stick with long-term.

What gives me hope is that AI is democratizing access to personalized health guidance. The kind of detailed analysis that used to require expensive specialists will be available through your phone. This means people in underserved communities can get the same quality of personalized advice as anyone else.

The goal isn't perfection—it's progress. AI helps you focus on the changes that will make the biggest difference for your health, whether that's losing 10 pounds or 100. Every small improvement in your health matters, and AI makes those improvements more achievable than ever before.

CHAPTER 6

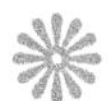

# DEMENTIA AND AI: PREVENTION, DETECTION, AND MANAGEMENT

Dementia is not one disease. It's a group of conditions that damage memory, thinking, and daily activities. It's something many of us fear most. Most people hear "dementia" and think Alzheimer's. They're right to focus there—it makes up 60–80% of all dementia cases. Vascular dementia is the second most common at 10–20%.

Alzheimer's mainly causes memory loss. People have the most trouble forming new memories. The disease creates sticky clumps called amyloid plaques in the brain. It also makes tangled fibers called tau proteins. Together, these slowly kill brain cells.

While scientists work on treatments for these proteins, research shows surprising diet findings. A major UK study of nearly 500,000 people found that eating unprocessed red meat may lower dementia risk by up to 30%, while processed meats like bacon and hot dogs may increase risk by up to 52% (Zhang et al., 2021). Low-carb, high-fat diets like the modified Atkins diet might also help. They give the brain ketones to use for energy when it can't use sugar properly (Brandt et al., 2019).

Vascular dementia happens when blood vessels in the brain get blocked or damaged. This often occurs after small strokes. It can also happen after years of high blood pressure or diabetes. Brain cells die when they don't get enough oxygen and nutrients. High-carb diets greatly increase the risk—people who eat lots of carbs have an 89% higher risk of dementia. Being overweight also raises risk. Extra weight causes inflammation and damages blood vessels throughout the body, including the brain. Unlike Alzheimer's, vascular dementia first affects thinking speed and problem-solving more than memory.

Other types are less common but still serious:

- **Lewy body dementia** (5–10% of cases): Protein clumps cause vivid hallucinations and sleep problems. People also have movement problems like those with Parkinson's disease.
- **Frontotemporal dementia** (5–10% of cases): This attacks the front and sides of the brain. It changes personality and behavior more than memory. People might become rude or lose empathy.
- **Parkinson's dementia** (2–5% of cases): Some people with Parkinson's disease develop this. They have movement problems such as tremor and shuffling gait, plus confusion and hallucinations.

While we don't fully understand what causes every type of dementia, we do know who's at risk. Age remains the strongest factor—your chances double every 5 years after 65. This affects millions of families, making it crucial to understand what we can and can't control about our risk. But here's the hopeful news: studies show we might prevent up to 40% of dementia cases through lifestyle changes (Livingston et al., 2020). This changes everything. Dementia isn't just fate. We can fight back, especially with AI tools that can catch it early.

## Role of Genetics in Dementia Risk

As we talked about in Chapter 2, your genes affect your chance of getting dementia. The *APOE* gene is the most important one. If you have the ε4 type, your risk goes up—but remember, having this gene doesn't mean you'll definitely develop dementia.

If you haven't had genetic testing yet (we covered this in Chapter 2), deciding whether to get tested can be hard, especially if dementia runs in your family. Tests still cost $100–200 from companies like 23andMe or Nebula Genomics. Getting your results can be scary, so talking to a genetic counselor helps.

Other genes besides *APOE* also matter. For Alzheimer's, these include *SORL1*, *CLU*, *PICALM*, and *TREM2*. For vascular dementia (when blood vessels in the brain get damaged), different genes like *MTHFR*, *NOTCH3*, and *ACE* play a role. These other genes don't affect your risk as much as *APOE* does.

### Joe's Fight Against Fate

Joe's story shows what it's like when bad genes meet family history. At 58, Joe had watched dementia destroy his family. His mom died from Alzheimer's at 71. His grandfather had a stroke at 55 and died from vascular dementia. Now Joe was having his own problems: getting confused, having trouble planning his day, and forgetting words.

When his gene test showed he had *APOE* ε4/ε4 (I explained this in Chapter 2), Joe was crushed. This gene doesn't just raise Alzheimer's risk. It also damages blood vessels and reduces blood flow to the brain, increasing the risk of vascular dementia—the same disease that killed his grandfather.

But Joe's story proves the main point from Chapter 2: your genes don't control everything. The Lancet Commission study from 2020 (Livingston et al., 2020) showed that healthy habits help even people with the worst genetic risks.

The *APOE* ε4 gene doesn't just raise Alzheimer's risk. It may also lead to vascular dementia. Studies show ε4 carriers have higher risk of heart disease and death. The gene speeds up blood vessel damage. It reduces blood flow to the brain.

Joe doesn't know something important. Vascular dementia has better treatments than Alzheimer's. Doctors can treat blood vessel problems. They control blood pressure and cholesterol. This can slow the disease and help people function longer. But first, Joe needs to see his doctor.

His friend Larry brought soup. He saw Joe's worried face. 'Got the results?' Larry asked.

'Yeah, it's bad,' Joe said quietly.

Larry was direct. 'Your genes are set, Joe. But you can still do something about it.'

Joe's cholesterol was sky-high. He ate lots of carbs and deli meats. He barely exercised. But Joe doesn't quit. A week later, he bought a smartwatch. He took a shaky 5-minute walk. His neighbor Mike saw him.

"Want to try some weights in my garage?" Mike asked. Joe shrugged.

"Why not?" That night, Joe lifted light weights—just a start. At dinner, he ate fewer fries. He savored each one like a small victory. The next day, he ordered salad instead of a burger.

"Becoming a rabbit, Joe?" the waitress joked.

"Gotta start somewhere," he smiled back.

It's not perfect. Change takes time. But his smartwatch reminds him to move. It tracks his sleep and meals. Small steps, Joe tells himself. He's pushing back against fate, one day at a time. For Joe, it's not just about beating the odds. It's about understanding his genes—a key piece in fighting dementia.

## Dementia Risk Across Different Communities

Research shows substantial variation in dementia risk factors and prevalence across different populations, making culturally informed AI approaches essential.

Black Americans face about one and a half times the rate of Alzheimer's disease as White Americans, with 14% of Black people over age 65 having Alzheimer's compared to 10% of White people (PBS NewsHour, 2023). While the *APOE* ε4 variant appears to have less impact in Black populations, other factors like cardiovascular disease and diabetes play more significant roles. Black Americans have diabetes rates of 12.1% compared to 6.9% for non-Hispanic White adults, and they experience hypertension rates that are among the highest in the world (Barnes & Bennett, 2014; CDC, 2024a).

Beyond these biological factors, Black communities often face socioeconomic and other barriers, including limited access to fresh foods, fewer safe spaces for exercise, and higher rates of conditions like stroke that increase dementia risk.

Hispanic Americans also have approximately one and a half times higher rates of Alzheimer's disease than non-Hispanic Whites, with research indicating that diabetes may be an especially important risk factor in this population (PBS

NewsHour, 2023). Language barriers in healthcare settings and lower rates of health insurance—approximately 19% of Hispanic Americans lack health coverage—can limit access to both preventive care and AI-based tools.

American Indians face unique challenges with limited research on prevalence and risk factors, complicated by historical trauma and significant limitations to access to healthcare. Traditional diets were dramatically altered by historical forces, replacing hunting and gathering with government-provided foods high in refined carbohydrates and unhealthy fats.

Asian Americans represent diverse populations with varying risk profiles. While overall dementia rates appear lower than among White Americans, studies indicate that the *APOE* ε4 variant may have stronger effects in East Asian populations (Huang et al., 2023). As we discussed in the previous chapter, Asian Americans tend to have smaller frames and may experience health complications at lower BMI thresholds—sometimes called skinny fat. This same pattern applies to dementia risk, requiring different assessment approaches for this population.

## Technology Access and Cultural Adaptation

The benefits of AI for dementia prevention and early detection vary significantly across different populations. AI-based dementia prevention tools must address both technological access and cultural appropriateness. This means developing tools that work on basic smartphones, providing content in multiple languages, respecting traditional healing practices alongside evidence-based medicine, and ensuring recommendations fit within cultural food preferences and family structures.

By acknowledging these differences and creating flexible approaches, AI can help reduce rather than reinforce health disparities in dementia prevention.

## How AI Can Help Lower Dementia Risk

AI offers powerful tools to help identify, monitor, and change dementia risk factors. Here's how AI can support prevention in key areas:

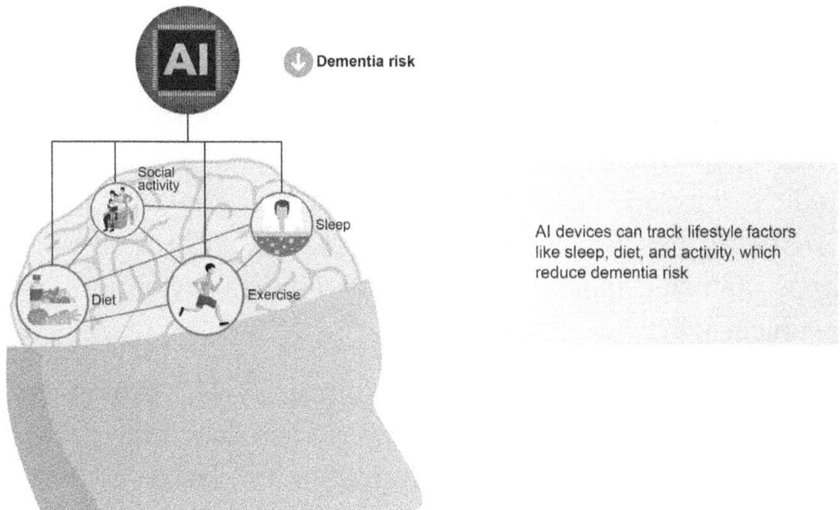
AI
Dementia risk
Social activity
Sleep
Diet
Exercise
AI devices can track lifestyle factors like sleep, diet, and activity, which reduce dementia risk

**Physical Activity and Exercise:** Regular exercise reduces dementia risk by 30–40%. AI wearables can track your daily activity, monitor your heart rate during workouts, give you personal recommendations based on your fitness level, and figure out what exercise routine you can stick with long-term. For current AI fitness devices and apps, ask an AI assistant: "What are the best AI fitness trackers and exercise apps?"

**Sleep Optimization:** Good sleep cuts dementia risk by 25–30%. AI sleep tools can monitor how long and how well you sleep, spot problems like sleep apnea that increase dementia risk, suggest the best bedtimes for you, and recommend changes to your bedroom environment. To find current sleep tracking options, ask: "What are the best AI sleep tracking devices and apps?"

**Nutrition and Diet:** Eating a Mediterranean or MIND diet can lower dementia risk by 20–30%. AI nutrition apps can identify foods from photos, suggest brain-healthy meals tailored to your needs, and create eating plans based on how your body responds to different foods.

**Cognitive Stimulation:** Mental activity builds your brain's resilience to damage. Studies show regular brain training may reduce dementia risk by 10–15%. Traditional options include crossword puzzles, chess, and card games. AI brain training apps offer specialized exercises for memory, attention, and problem-solving.

**Cardiovascular Health Monitoring:** Type 2 diabetes and high blood pressure significantly increase dementia risk. AI health monitoring can track your blood pressure patterns, monitor blood sugar levels, spot early warning signs of heart problems, and help you stick to your medications. Managing these factors in midlife can reduce dementia risk by up to 35%.

**Early Detection Through AI:** AI can spot early brain changes years before symptoms appear. Some companies offer whole-body scans that include the brain, while digital cognitive tests can track subtle changes in your thinking over time. Ask your local imaging center if they offer AI-enhanced brain scans, as this technology can improve detection by 15–20%.

One important note from medical research: if you add up all these percentages, it looks like you could eliminate dementia risk entirely—maybe even prevent it more than 100%!

Unfortunately, that's not how it works. These risk factors overlap and interact with each other in complex ways. For example, exercise improves sleep, which helps cardiovascular health, which affects brain health—so the benefits get counted multiple times. This is called the "prevention paradox" or overlapping risk reduction.

The reality? Even with perfect healthy living, you can reduce your dementia risk by about 40–60% from your baseline, according to the Lancet Commission (2020). That's still huge—imagine cutting your risk in half!—but it's not a guarantee. Your genes, age, and factors we don't yet understand still play a role. Think of it like wearing a seatbelt: it dramatically reduces your risk of dying in a car accident but doesn't eliminate it completely. The good news is that every healthy change you make counts, even if the math doesn't add up the way you'd expect.

For current AI tools in any of these areas, ask an AI assistant: "What are the best AI tools for dementia prevention?"

### Joe's Ongoing Journey

After 6 months of implementing AI-guided lifestyle changes, Joe has made remarkable progress. Joe's smartwatch tracks his 30-minute daily walks and three weekly workouts. His sleep quality has improved from 68% to 82% according to his Oura Ring, and his diet app shows he's following a Mediterranean eating pattern 70% of the time.

Most importantly, his quarterly cognitive assessment scores have remained stable, providing reassurance that his efforts are making a difference. Joe can't change his *APOE* gene, but his AI coach says lifestyle changes cut his dementia risk by about 30%.

"It's not about fighting my genes," Joe explains, "It's about giving my brain the best chance possible."

Joe's case illustrates the potential of AI to transform dementia prevention from abstract recommendations to personalized, actionable strategies that can meaningfully reduce risk—even for those with significant genetic predisposition.

## Key Takeaways

- Dementia risk is influenced by both genetic and lifestyle factors, with up to 40% of cases potentially preventable through modifiable risk factor management.
- AI technologies provide powerful tools for personalized risk assessment, early detection, and lifestyle modification across multiple domains, including exercise, nutrition, sleep, cognitive training, and cardiovascular health.
- Cultural factors significantly influence both dementia risk and access to AI-based prevention tools, requiring culturally informed and equitable approaches.
- Early detection through AI-enhanced cognitive assessments, speech analysis, and digital biomarkers may identify cognitive changes years before clinical diagnosis.
- Early implementation of AI-guided prevention strategies may substantially reduce risk, even for individuals with high genetic predisposition.

While no approach can guarantee prevention, the combination of early detection and personalized intervention offers the best current strategy for reducing dementia risk and extending cognitive health.

## Looking Forward

Dementia research is accelerating at a pace I've never seen before, and AI is at the center of these breakthroughs. We're moving from a time when dementia felt like an inevitable fate to one where prevention and early intervention offer real hope.

In the coming years, AI will help us predict dementia risk decades before symptoms appear. Your smartphone might detect subtle changes in your speech patterns or walking rhythm that suggest brain changes are beginning. Smart home devices could notice that you're having more trouble with complex tasks, prompting early intervention when it can do the most good.

What's most promising is how AI is helping us understand that dementia isn't one disease but many different conditions requiring different approaches. Soon, AI will help create personalized prevention plans based on your specific risk factors—whether that's genetics, sleep patterns, cardiovascular health, or environmental exposures.

The lifestyle changes we know help prevent dementia—exercise, good sleep, social connection, mental stimulation—will become easier to maintain with AI coaching. Instead of vague advice to "stay active," you'll get specific guidance on the types of exercise that benefit your brain most, tailored to your abilities and preferences.

For families already affected by dementia, AI is creating tools to help maintain dignity and connection longer. Smart home systems can provide gentle reminders and safety monitoring without feeling intrusive. Communication aids can help preserve relationships even as memory fades.

Joe's story shows what's possible when we combine genetic knowledge with AI-guided lifestyle changes. While we can't change our genes, we can change how those genes express themselves. The future of dementia care isn't about accepting decline—it's about fighting back with science, technology, and hope.

CHAPTER 7

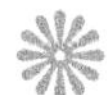

# BREAST CANCER AND AI: HOW TECHNOLOGY CAN HELP PREVENT AND TREAT

## What You Really Need to Know About Breast Cancer

Breast cancer touches many lives—about 1 in 8 women will face it during their lifetime. That is scary, but here's the good news: When caught early, the 5-year survival rate is an amazing 99–100% (American Cancer Society, 2024; National Cancer Institute, 2024). Over the past few decades, we've made incredible progress. Since the 1990s, deaths from breast cancer have dropped by 40%. This happened thanks to better screening, improved treatments, and women standing up for their health.

Most importantly, this progress came from women helping women. Sisters, mothers, and daughters turned their grief and fear into action. They organized walks and runs that raised billions for research. They demanded better treatments and earlier detection. They pushed Congress for funding. Organizations like Susan G. Komen, founded by a woman who lost her sister to breast cancer, changed how we fight this disease. Women researchers fought for careers in oncology when few were welcome. Women advocates made pink ribbons a symbol everyone recognizes. This isn't just medical progress—it's what happens when women refuse to accept "that's just how it is" and demand better for each other.

So, what exactly is breast cancer? It happens when cells in your breast start growing out of control. Most cases begin in the milk ducts—the tubes that carry milk if you've had a baby. Many breast cancers are fueled by hormones like estrogen that your body makes naturally. This actually gives doctors a way to fight back using medicines that can block these hormones. Plus, your immune system is already working to spot and destroy cancer cells before they become a problem. New treatments called immune therapy make your natural defenses even stronger.

Some risk factors come from your family history, while others are things you can change, like how much you exercise or drink alcohol. Your genes also contain crucial clues about your breast cancer risk. I believe genetic testing should be available to every woman who wants it.

Testing has become more affordable with multiple options. Targeted cancer gene panels cost $200–500 and focus specifically on *BRCA* and related genes. Whole genome sequencing examines all your DNA—labs can read your genetic code 30 times for around $300–500, or 100 times for $500–1,000 (more readings mean fewer errors and more reliable results). Research labs like Myriad and Ambry specialize in medical-grade *BRCA* testing with clinical oversight. Premium services like New Amsterdam Genomics ($3,000+) provide the most thorough analysis, lifetime reanalysis as genetic science improves, and direct access to genetic counselors. Many of these options are now affordable enough to pay out of pocket for this one-time test that provides lifetime information.

There are genes called *BRCA1* and *BRCA2* that, when changed or mutated, greatly increase breast cancer risk—up to 72% by age 80 (Kuchenbaecker et al., 2017). Here's what surprises many people: About half of women with these dangerous gene changes don't have any family history that would trigger insurance coverage for testing. Without testing, they'd never know they were at high risk.

While current medical guidelines limit testing to women with certain risk factors—largely because of cost concerns—I believe broader access to genetic testing could save lives by finding these hidden risks. Talk to your doctor about whether genetic testing makes sense for you and know that you have options even if insurance won't cover it.

The exciting part? Research shows that smart lifestyle changes can cut your risk by up to 50%. If you have a higher genetic risk, adding extra screening can lower it even more, sometimes by as much as 80%!

## Breast Cancer Risk Across Different Communities

Different women face different challenges when it comes to breast cancer prevention, detection, and treatment. Let's look at how AI can help address these gaps for women from various backgrounds.

White women have the highest breast cancer rates—about 141 out of every 100,000 women each year, which works out to that familiar 1 in 8 lifetime risk (Hirko et al., 2022). Here's an important detail: Most breast cancers in White women (about 80%) have hormone receptors, which is actually good news because it means these cancers often respond well to hormone-blocking treatments. The typical age when White women are diagnosed is around 65, though of course it can happen earlier or later (Giaquinto et al., 2022).

Black women face unique and serious challenges with breast cancer. While they get breast cancer less often—about 119 out of every 100,000 women each year—they're 40% more likely to die from it than White women (Siegel et al., 2023). Why this terrible gap? It's both biological and social. Black women are twice as likely to get triple-negative breast cancer, a particularly aggressive type. About 21% of Black women with breast cancer have this hard-to-treat form, compared to only 10% of White women (Hirko et al., 2022). Studies also suggest that harmful *BRCA* gene changes might affect Black women more severely (Churpek et al., 2015).

On top of these biological challenges, many Black women face real barriers to getting quality care. Many Black neighborhoods have fewer doctors, meaning ridiculously long wait times just to get an appointment. Without insurance, a mammogram can cost hundreds of dollars. When the nearest breast imaging center is an hour away and you don't have a car, or when you can't take time off work without losing pay, getting screened becomes nearly impossible. Add to this the medical mistrust rooted in historical injustices—generations of discrimination that make some women hesitant to seek help even when they can (Molina et al., 2015). These barriers pile up, making everything worse.

Hispanic women develop breast cancer even less often—about 90 out of every 100,000 women each year, compared to 141 for White women (Hirko et al., 2022). But here's the problem: when Hispanic women do get breast cancer, it's often found later, when it's harder to treat. Why? Many Hispanic women also face real barriers to healthcare. They might not have insurance, live far from cancer centers, or face language barriers that make it hard to navigate the healthcare system. These delays in diagnosis mean Hispanic women often need more aggressive treatment and may have worse outcomes, even though they get breast cancer less often.

Asian and Pacific Islander women have lower breast cancer rates too—about 97 out of every 100,000 women (Hirko et al., 2022). However, their experience with the disease has important differences. They're more likely to develop breast cancer before age 50, when many women haven't started getting regular mammograms yet. Many Asian women also have dense breast tissue—imagine trying to spot a snowball in a snowstorm on an X-ray. This makes mammograms less reliable for them. These factors mean Asian women might need different screening approaches, starting earlier or using additional tests like ultrasound, MRI, or molecular breast imaging (MBI).

American Indian and Alaska Native women have the lowest breast cancer rates—about 78 out of every 100,000 women, compared to 141 for White women (Islami et al., 2022). But lower rates don't mean fewer problems. Many Native women live far from cancer centers, sometimes hundreds of miles from the nearest mammogram machine. Some reservations have limited healthcare services, and traveling for treatment can mean long trips that take women away from work and family. These distance and resource barriers mean that when Native women do get breast cancer, it's often caught later, making it harder to treat successfully.

### Changing the Game: AI and Prevention

Testing your genes creates millions of data points—far too many for any doctor to analyze. AI can scan through this genetic information in seconds, flagging mutations like

*BRCA* that might spell trouble. It doesn't stop there—AI can combine your genetic information with other factors like age, weight, and lifestyle habits to calculate your personal risk score. This powerful knowledge lets you and your doctor create a screening plan based on your actual risk, not general guidelines.

Your personal risk level should guide how often you get screened. Mammograms are typically recommended yearly, starting at age 40 for women at average risk. But for women between 40 and 50 without extra risk factors, mammograms do not always provide much benefit. Studies show they only slightly lower the death rate in this group, perhaps helping just 1 or 2 women out of 1,000. False alarms are common too, leading to unnecessary worry and extra tests.

But if your risk is higher—because you have a *BRCA* mutation or close relatives who were diagnosed with breast cancer at a young age—mammograms become much more valuable and should start earlier, sometimes at age 25 or 30. Your screening program should be personalized.

## AI Makes Screening Smarter

AI is changing how mammograms work. Traditional mammogram reading depends on doctors who, while skilled, are human and can miss subtle signs or flag normal tissue as suspicious. AI systems can now analyze mammogram images, comparing patterns against millions of other images with incredible accuracy. These systems can sometimes spot early signs of cancer that human eyes might miss, catching cancers much earlier than they would otherwise be found (McKinney et al., 2020). It's like having an extremely experienced colleague double-check every mammogram, one who has learned from reviewing millions of cases.

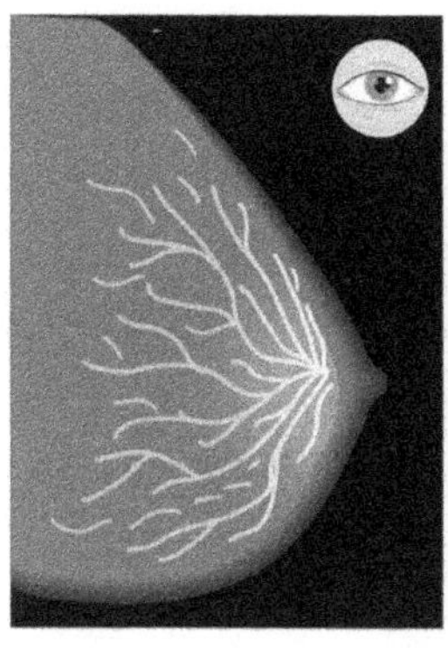

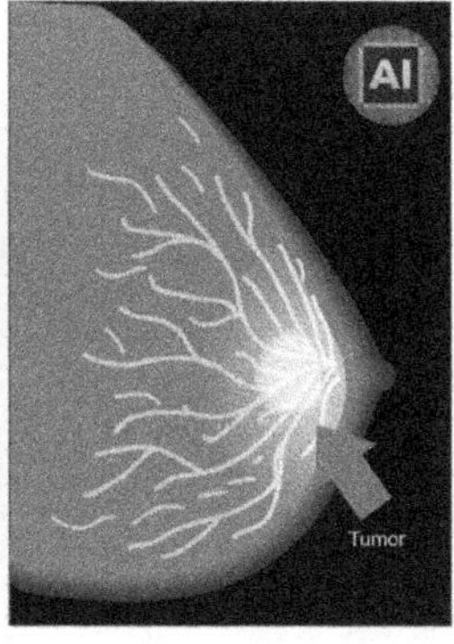


AI can spot patterns that remain undetected by human eyes and support early detection of tumors in dense breast cancer tissues

For women with dense breast tissue (about 40% of women), mammograms can be less effective—again, it's like looking for a snowball in a snowstorm. This is where AI really helps by highlighting subtle patterns that might indicate cancer. AI can also suggest when additional tests like an ultrasound or MRI would be beneficial, especially for women with dense breasts or breast implants or who are at higher risk.

Studies show that AI can reduce false negatives (missed cancers) by up to 20% and false positives (unnecessary callbacks) by up to 30%. Take Carmen, whose routine mammogram looked normal to the doctor. However, the AI system flagged a tiny area of concern, leading to an ultrasound that found a small tumor that might have been missed for another year. Because it was caught so early, Carmen needed less aggressive treatment and was cured.

## AI and Treatment

If you do face a breast cancer diagnosis, AI becomes even more valuable. Here's how:

AI helps doctors choose the most effective treatment plan by analyzing the genetic makeup of your specific cancer. Not all breast cancers are the same; they have different mutations and respond differently to treatments. AI can match the profile of your cancer with thousands of similar cases, predicting which treatments worked best for patients like you.

During chemotherapy, AI can monitor how your tumor is responding and suggest adjustments to your treatment if needed. Some women get more chemo than they need, while others don't get enough. AI helps personalize the dose, minimizing side effects while maximizing effectiveness.

For surgery, AI can assist in planning the procedure, helping surgeons remove all the cancer while preserving as much healthy tissue as possible. This is especially important for breast-saving surgeries, where the goal is to maintain appearance while ensuring all cancer cells are removed.

Even after treatment, AI keeps working for you. Wearable devices can track subtle changes in your body that might indicate a recurrence, allowing for earlier intervention if needed. AI can also predict your risk of recurrence, helping determine how frequently you need follow-up visits and scans.

### Taking Action: What You Can Do Today

You don't need to be a tech expert to benefit from AI in breast cancer prevention and treatment. Here are practical steps you can take:

**Learn your family history.** Talk to relatives on both sides of your family about any cancer diagnoses, especially breast, ovarian, pancreatic, or prostate cancers. These cancers can be linked together by the same gene changes—particularly *BRCA1* and *BRCA2* mutations—so having one type in your family may increase your risk for others. This is key for all women but especially important for Black women, who may have higher genetic risks.

**Consider genetic testing.** If you have a family history of these cancers, ask your doctor about *BRCA* testing—targeted cancer gene panels typically cost $200–500, or specialized research labs like Myriad and Ambry offer medical-grade analysis. Even without family history, whole genome sequencing provides valuable information about many health risks, including breast cancer. Basic whole genome sequencing (where labs read your DNA 30 times) costs $300–500, while more thorough testing (100 readings for higher accuracy) runs $500–1,000. This is particularly important for Asian women, who may have "silent" genetic risks without a family history.

**Know your breast density.** After your mammogram, ask about your breast density and whether additional screening might be helpful. Dense breast tissue makes mammograms less effective and may require extra testing like an ultrasound or MRI.

**Use online risk calculators.** Tools like the Tyrer-Cuzick model (available on websites like MagView or Ikonopedia) use AI to estimate your breast cancer risk based on multiple factors.

**Ask about AI-enhanced mammograms.** When scheduling your mammogram, ask if the facility uses AI to help interpret results. Push for this technology, especially if you live in an area with limited healthcare resources.

**Make lifestyle changes.** Even with genetic risks, healthy choices matter. Don't drink alcohol, or if you do, limit it to less than one drink per day. Maintain a healthy weight, stay physically active, and eat plenty of fruits, vegetables, and whole grains. These changes can cut your risk by up to 50% for women of all backgrounds.

**Be your own advocate.** If you notice changes in your breasts—like a lump, skin changes, nipple discharge, or new pain—don't wait for your next scheduled mammogram. See your doctor promptly. Think of Diane. She had no family history of breast cancer but decided to get genetic testing anyway. When AI analysis of her genes revealed a *BRCA* mutation, she started getting MRIs yearly and made lifestyle changes like exercising more and limiting alcohol. So far, she remains cancer-free. Her story shows how AI technology can help you understand your risk and take action, even when your family history doesn't suggest a problem.

## Looking Forward

Breast cancer care is entering an era that would have seemed like science fiction just a few years ago. We're moving toward a future where prevention isn't just about lifestyle changes but about understanding your personal risk at the molecular level and acting on that knowledge before cancer ever appears.

AI is transforming every aspect of breast cancer care. Soon, your annual mammogram will be read by AI systems that can spot cancers years before they become visible to human eyes. These same systems will analyze your breast density, family history, and genetic profile to create screening schedules designed specifically for you—not generic guidelines applied to everyone.

For women at high risk, AI will monitor subtle changes in blood tests, analyzing patterns that might indicate cancer is developing. Wearable devices might detect metabolic shifts or immune system changes that serve as early warning signals. This isn't about living in fear—it's about having powerful allies watching out for your health.

What gives me the most hope is how AI is making personalized medicine accessible to everyone. The genetic testing and risk analysis that once required expensive specialists will soon be available through your phone. This means women in rural areas or underserved communities can access the same cutting-edge prevention strategies as anyone else.

Treatment is becoming more precise too. AI will analyze your tumor's genetic fingerprint to predict exactly which treatments will work best for your specific cancer, minimizing side effects while maximizing effectiveness. Recovery monitoring through AI will catch complications early and help optimize your healing process.

The goal isn't just surviving breast cancer—it's preventing it entirely when possible, catching it early when prevention isn't enough, and treating it with such precision that it becomes a manageable chapter in your life rather than a defining crisis. AI is making all of this possible, one breakthrough at a time.

CHAPTER 8

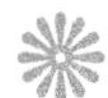

# COLON CANCER AND AI: YOUR PARTNER FOR PREVENTION, DETECTION, AND TREATMENT

Colon cancer is serious business, ranking third in worldwide cancer cases and second in U.S. cancer deaths. I've seen it blindside patients and families with late-stage diagnoses that could have been caught earlier. The cancer begins silently as polyps, small mushroom-like growths in your colon that can become cancerous if left alone. Finding and removing these polyps through screening can lower your risk by up to 80%, but many people skip this vital step due to fear, inconvenience, or simple lack of awareness. Colonoscopy is still the best way to find and remove these polyps before they become dangerous, but it takes preparation, sedation, and time away from work. This is where AI comes in—not to replace your doctor but to help spot problems early, prevent issues where possible, and improve treatment when needed. The goal is to help you live well, not just survive.

AI is already making a difference, and what's coming next is impressive. Picture your phone warning you about risky foods from a simple photo, a genetic test showing your personal risk level, or stool tests becoming so easy they're just part of your yearly routine. For the most serious cases—colon cancer that has spread beyond the colon—AI is already finding better drugs with fewer side effects.

## The Basics of Colon Cancer

Colon cancer grows in your large intestine, often without any warning signs until it's advanced. Polyps are the warning flags—some harmless, others precancerous. Your risk goes up with processed meat consumption, a low-fiber diet, lack of exercise, smoking, certain genes, and age (especially after 45).

However, there has been a recent and significant rise in colorectal cancer among people under 50, with a cumulative increase of about 50% since the 1990s (Siegel et al., 2023). Researchers believe this increase may be caused by several factors (in order of importance): rising obesity rates, increased consumption of processed foods and sugary drinks, sedentary lifestyles, and changes in the gut bacteria (aka microbiome) due to antibiotic use and altered diets (Akimoto et al., 2021).

Let me tell you about James, a 52-year-old patient who assumed he was safe from colon cancer. After all, nobody in his family had it, and screening usually starts at 50. He would have waited even longer, but something unexpected changed his mind. When an AI diet tracking app analyzed his high processed meat intake along with his age and calculated his personal colon cancer risk as elevated, he scheduled a screening immediately. Doctors found and removed three precancerous polyps. "That app probably saved my life," he said. "I had no symptoms at all.

## Colon Cancer Across Different Communities

Colon cancer affects different communities in different ways, and access to AI solutions varies too. White Americans have colorectal cancer incidence rates of approximately 35.8 per 100,000 people, with a lifetime risk of about 1 in 24 for men and 1 in 26 for women (American Cancer Society, 2023).

Black Americans face 40% higher rates of colon cancer at 40.4 per 100,000, with diagnoses often coming at later stages (Augustus & Ellis, 2018). AI tools for diet tracking and genetic risk assessment could help reduce this gap by 20–30%. But as with other cancers and diseases, historical distrust of medical institutions creates barriers. Programs that pair AI tools with trusted community health workers show the most promise.

Hispanic Americans have colorectal cancer rates of 32.3 per 100,000, which is actually lower than White Americans but still represents a significant health burden (Siegel et al., 2023). Despite having fewer high-risk genetic markers, they often face delayed diagnoses due to lower screening rates (Carethers, 2021). Family-centered care traditions can sometimes delay formal screening. Spanish-language apps with family-oriented messaging could increase screening rates by 15–25%.

American Indians and Alaska Natives experience colorectal cancer rates of 25.7 per 100,000, lower than White Americans. However, they face the highest mortality rates of all groups due to rural isolation and limited internet access that restrict their use of AI tools (Melkonian et al., 2019). Solutions that work offline and respect traditional healing practices show the most potential for these communities.

Asian Americans have the lowest colorectal cancer rates among major racial groups at 28.6 per 100,000—about 20% lower than White Americans—and higher technology adoption rates. However, cultural barriers that include feelings of embarrassment and shame around screening procedures can delay needed testing (Ma et al., 2009). Privacy-focused tools with culturally sensitive education could increase screening rates by 20–30% in these communities.

### Prevention: AI as Your Personal Health Coach

AI is transforming how we prevent colon cancer through personalized advice tailored just for you. Take a photo of your lunch—like a bacon cheeseburger—and AI can instantly spot the processed meat, which studies link to a 20–30% higher cancer risk. Apps like Cronometer AI can analyze weeks of your eating patterns and suggest specific changes based on what you actually like to eat. Instead of general advice like "eat more fiber," AI might suggest swapping your breakfast bacon for turkey bacon or recommend high-fiber foods you've enjoyed before.

Some advanced apps even track your location and alert you to environmental risks, while barcode-scanning tools can check your household products for potential cancer-causing chemicals. These tools are remarkably cost-effective—a $5–10 monthly subscription could potentially prevent cancer.

The economic case for AI makes sense. AI diet apps costing $5–10 monthly could reduce cancer risk by 15–20%, preventing treatments that cost over $100,000. AI-enhanced tests may add $100–200 to the procedure but catch more polyps, preventing expensive late-stage treatments. For treatment, spending $5,000–10,000 on AI analysis could prevent $20,000 or more in complications.

### Detection: Finding Cancer Earlier and More Accurately

Early detection is where AI truly shines. New systems like GI Genius (approved in 2021) work alongside your doctor during a colonoscopy, pointing out polyps that might be missed by the human eye alone (Wallace et al., 2022). Studies show these systems find 10–15% more polyps (Repici et al., 2020), which means removing dangerous growths before they turn into cancer. Before scheduling a colonoscopy, ask if they use AI-enhanced equipment.

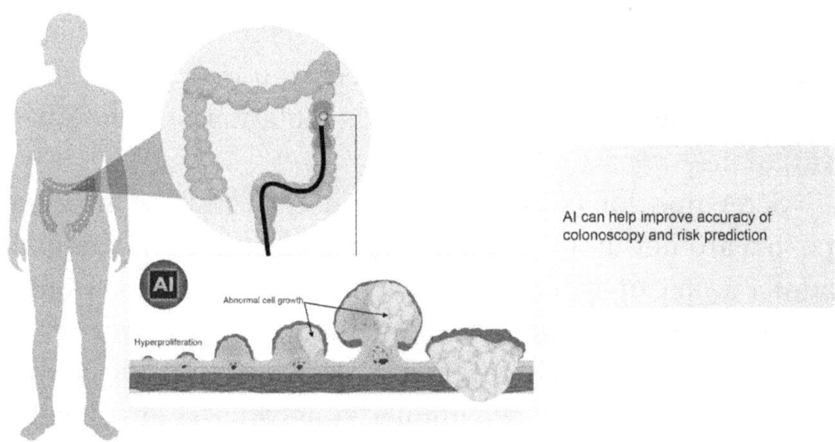
AI
Abnormal cell growth
Hyperproliferation
AI can help improve accuracy of colonoscopy and risk prediction

Colonoscopies have major advantages. While Cologuard (discussed below) detects about 43% of precancerous polyps, colonoscopies can find about 95% of them. More importantly, during a colonoscopy, doctors can remove polyps immediately—if Cologuard finds something suspicious, you'll still need a colonoscopy to remove it. Colonoscopies are also better at finding flat lesions, which can sometimes develop into aggressive cancers.

Stool tests are getting better, too. Current tests like Cologuard look for cancer markers in your stool with about 95% accuracy for detecting early cancers. This makes it a good option for people who can't have colonoscopies due to health issues or age concerns or who strongly prefer not to have one.

However, Cologuard is not a replacement for a colonoscopy, which remains the most accurate test. The good news is that most insurance plans now cover Cologuard at no cost for eligible patients aged 45–75, and follow-up colonoscopies are also covered without copays.

AI is also making genetic testing more useful. Rather than just checking for a few specific gene mutations, AI analyzes your entire genetic profile and understands how different genetic factors work together to affect your risk. It can tell the difference between truly dangerous mutations and harmless variations.

Screening for colon cancer is unique because so many people are hesitant to do it or refuse—about 40% of eligible adults aren't up to date with screening. In general, women get suggested mammograms, and former smokers get chest X-rays without much resistance. However, having a tube inserted through your rectum under anesthesia or collecting your stool and sending it in the mail is not appealing. Like with most medical tests, I have done both and can honestly say the experiences are not bad and worth it—nowhere near as bad as imagined—and not painful. Pleasant would be a sales pitch.

I wrestled with whether or how to write about a third option because at present it doesn't work as well as the other two for colon cancer. Again, colon cancer is slow growing (over a couple to a few years) and curable if caught early—deadly if not. But if you just won't get a colonoscopy or a Cologuard stool test, there are new blood test options.

Blood tests for colon cancer have arrived, making screening as simple as a regular blood draw. Guardant Health's Shield test got FDA approval in 2024 and costs about $895, detecting colon cancer from a simple blood sample. GRAIL's

Galleri test goes even further, screening for over 50 types of cancer from one blood sample for around $950, though it's not yet approved by the FDA for colon cancer specifically. Exact Sciences (makers of Cologuard) is developing their own blood test called CancerGuard. While these blood tests aren't as accurate as colonoscopy yet—Shield catches about 83% of colon cancers compared to colonoscopy's 95%—they're a game-changer for people who refuse traditional screening. Check with your insurance—many don't yet cover these newer blood tests. Researchers are also working on experimental sensors that might detect early cancer signs in your sweat or breath, though these are still years away.

### Using AI Tools for Early Detection and Monitoring

Wearable devices and smartphones are becoming valuable tools in colon cancer prevention and early detection. While no smartwatch can directly detect colon cancer yet, several provide data that might alert you to warning signs like fatigue and shortness of breath during exercise, unexplained weight loss, changes in heart rate patterns that could indicate anemia from internal bleeding, or disrupted sleep patterns that might signal discomfort or pain.

Smartphone apps add another layer of protection. Screening reminder apps like HealthyYou can integrate with your health record to determine your personal screening schedule based on risk factors and then provide timely reminders. Symptom tracker apps can analyze combinations of symptoms that individually might seem minor but together suggest a need for medical attention.

One of AI's most powerful applications is personalizing the interpretation of your routine lab work. Rather than relying solely on population-based "normal" ranges, AI establishes your personal baseline. For example, if your hemoglobin typically runs around 14 g/dL, a drop to 12 g/dL—still technically within the "normal" range—could indicate blood loss, potentially from a colorectal tumor. AI systems flag these personal deviations when standard lab reports wouldn't. They can spot declining iron stores (measured by ferritin) months before noticeable hemoglobin drops and detect subtle elevations in inflammatory markers that might warrant investigation.

## Genetic Risk Analysis: From Commercial Testing to Whole Genome AI

Modern genetic testing with AI interpretation provides a much more precise picture of your cancer risk than family history alone. Commercial tests now screen for key genes linked to colon cancer risk, such as *APC* (associated with familial adenomatous polyposis, with 50–70% lifetime risk from a single mutation) and *MLH1/MSH2* (associated with Lynch Syndrome, with 50–80% lifetime risk).

What makes AI special is how it interprets these results. Rather than simply noting whether a mutation is present, AI systems analyze exactly where the mutation occurs in the gene, how it might interact with other genes, and how your lifestyle factors might increase or decrease your risk. AI can distinguish between truly dangerous mutations and harmless variations—important since up to 40% of genetic findings are initially classified as "uncertain significance."

The cutting edge is whole genome analysis with AI interpretation. This examines your entire genetic code, not just a few selected genes. AI checks your full DNA report to spot colon cancer risks, suggesting how often you need screenings.

Those with the highest risk might need a colonoscopy every year to protect them from colon cancer.

Based on this comprehensive genetic assessment, AI creates personalized screening recommendations. If you have high-risk mutations like those causing Lynch syndrome, you might need annual colonoscopies starting at age 25. With moderate risk factors, you might need colonoscopies every 2–3 years starting at age 40–45.

This personalized approach makes economic sense too—the one-time cost of comprehensive genetic analysis ($500–1,000) prevents years of unnecessary yearly screenings for low-risk individuals while ensuring high-risk patients get the close monitoring they need.

For those prioritizing cancer prevention over cost, consider more frequent screening than standard guidelines suggest. You might get colonoscopies every 5 years or add Cologuard tests between colonoscopies. Why? Because the standard 10-year colonoscopy interval is based on what's cost-effective for the healthcare system, not what's best for preventing cancer.

Here's what you should know: Studies show that 16–18% of colon cancers show up within 5 years of a clean colonoscopy (Changchien et al., 2014; Eren et al., 2012). Most of these cancers appear in the first 3 years. While most colon cancers grow slowly, some aggressive types can develop and become deadly within 3–5 years.

The current guidelines say people at average risk should get a colonoscopy every 10 years starting at age 45, or Cologuard stool tests every 3 years (Shaukat et al., 2021). These recommendations balance cancer prevention with healthcare costs. But if you want maximum protection and can afford it, more frequent screening makes sense.

## Treatment: AI-Enhanced Approaches for Better Outcomes

For those diagnosed with colon cancer, AI is changing how treatment works, especially for advanced cases. **If you receive a cancer diagnosis, ask your doctor about genetic testing of your tumor that uses AI to find the best treatment for you.** AI can analyze your tumor's genetic profile alongside thousands of similar cases to predict which drugs will work best for your specific cancer type.

Smart dosing systems can recommend medication schedules that keep drugs effective while reducing side effects based on your age, metabolism, and other health conditions. For complex cases, AI can help determine the best order of treatments—when to use chemotherapy, immunotherapy, or targeted therapy for maximum benefit (Liao et al., 2023).

AI can spot subtle patterns in tumor genetics that predict which patients will respond to immunotherapy drugs like nivolumab and ipilimumab. For targeted therapies, AI mapping of tumor DNA can match patients with specific drugs that work best for their particular cancer mutations. Beyond your immediate treatment team, resources like Cancer Commons use AI to match patients with clinical trials for their specific type of cancer—something worth exploring if standard treatments aren't working as hoped.

AI has also improved planning for chemotherapy and radiation therapy, making it easier to evaluate how well treatments are working (Yin et al., 2023). Many hospitals now offer programs that use AI to monitor for side effects from home. These systems can catch problems early before they get serious, giving you and your care team time to adjust your treatment.

Recent studies show that AI-driven treatment plans reduced side effects by about 25% while improving effectiveness by approximately 15%. This means less suffering and more quality time for patients, especially those with advanced disease.

## AI as Your Medical Literature Helper

One of AI's most valuable but overlooked roles is making complex medical research accessible to patients. Medical literature on colon cancer is vast and often contradictory—over 15,000 new studies are published each year, making it impossible even for specialists to stay current. AI systems can analyze thousands of studies at once, translate dense medical terminology into everyday language, and highlight findings most relevant to your specific situation.

Several AI tools now provide this research interpretation service. Scite summarizes recent research in plain language and shows whether studies support or contradict medical claims. Elicit answers specific medical questions by synthesizing findings across studies. Research Rabbit monitors new publications in areas of interest and alerts you when relevant studies appear.

For colon cancer specifically, these tools can help you understand the evidence behind different screening methods, how your personal risk factors might warrant deviating from standard guidelines, emerging prevention and detection technologies, and the real-world effectiveness of treatments.

This knowledge can be lifesaving. Understanding that some fast-growing colon cancers can develop between standard screenings might prompt you to discuss additional stool-based testing with your doctor, potentially catching a cancer that would otherwise be missed.

## Taking Action: Your Personal AI Colon Cancer Prevention Toolkit

**First, get digitally equipped.** Set up an Apple Health or Google Fit account to centralize your health data. Consider investing in a quality wearable with HRV tracking ($150–350) and download a comprehensive health tracking app with AI capabilities ($0–10/month).

**Next, establish your baselines (one at a time is fine).** Export at least 2 years of previous lab results to an AI health platform. Track at least 30 days of continuous HRV and activity data. Log your food intake for 2 weeks to establish dietary patterns.

**Set up smart screening protocols.** Use a screening reminder app that accounts for your personal risk factors. Consider genetic testing: targeted cancer gene panels cost $200–500, whole genome sequencing runs $300–1,000 (depending on whether the lab reads your DNA 30 or 100 times), and premium services with genetic counseling start around $3,000. You don't need family history to benefit—choose the option that fits your budget and how comprehensive you want the information. Configure lab tracking to alert you to personalized deviations.

**Enhance your conventional screening.** When scheduling a colonoscopy, specifically request AI-assisted technology to increase polyp detection by 10–15%. Ask your provider to compare your current lab tests against your personal history, not just reference ranges. Consider annual stool DNA tests between colonoscopies if you're at elevated risk.

**Monitor specific health signals.** Track hemoglobin, ferritin, and inflammatory markers annually. Set alerts for unexplained weight loss (more than 5% in 6 months). Monitor any persistent changes in bowel habits using a dedicated app.

**If diagnosed,** request genomic tumor testing with AI analysis to identify optimal treatment. Use AI platforms like Cancer Commons to identify clinical trials matching your specific cancer profile. Consider remote monitoring programs that use AI to detect treatment side effects early.

**Stay informed** by setting Google Scholar alerts for new AI and colon cancer research, and joining smart patient communities like Smart Patients or PatientsLikeMe that filter the latest advances.

By combining these AI tools with regular medical care, you can take a more active role in protecting yourself from colon cancer. Technology doesn't replace doctors or eliminate the need for healthy lifestyle choices, but it does give you powerful new ways to prevent, detect, and fight this common but dangerous disease.

## Looking Forward

Colon cancer prevention is about to become much more personal and effective. We're moving from a world of one-size-fits-all screening schedules to precisely tailored approaches based on your individual risk factors, lifestyle, and genetic makeup.

AI is revolutionizing how we think about colon cancer risk. Soon, your smartphone camera will analyze your meals and warn you about dietary patterns that increase cancer risk, while genetic testing will reveal whether you need more frequent screening or can safely follow standard guidelines. Smart toilets—already being developed—will analyze your stool for early cancer markers, turning every bathroom visit into a screening opportunity.

The colonoscopy itself is becoming more accurate with AI assistance. These systems can spot polyps that human eyes might miss and predict which ones are most likely to become cancerous, allowing doctors to focus their attention where it matters most. For people who can't or won't have colonoscopies, the new blood tests that just hit the market can detect colon cancer from a simple blood draw. The technology is advancing quickly—these tests didn't even exist for consumers 5 years ago, and they're getting more accurate with every update.

AI is making prevention strategies work with your real life. Instead of generic advice to "eat more fiber," AI will suggest specific foods you actually enjoy that also reduce your cancer risk. It will identify your personal trigger times for poor food choices and offer alternatives that fit your schedule and preferences.

For those facing a colon cancer diagnosis, AI is creating treatment plans that are uniquely effective for your specific tumor type. Side effects are becoming more manageable as AI helps doctors adjust doses and timing based on how your body responds to treatment.

The future of colon cancer isn't about fear—it's about knowledge, early action, and treatments so effective that cancer becomes a manageable condition rather than a life-threatening crisis. AI is making this future possible by turning complex medical knowledge into simple, actionable steps you can take today.

CHAPTER 9

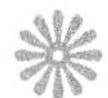

# LUNG CANCER AND AI: YOUR ALLY IN PREVENTION AND EARLY DETECTION

Lung cancer might not come to mind when you think of AI, but technology can really help here. Your lungs work hard, pulling oxygen from each breath into your blood. Inside, airways spread like tree branches. Tiny hairs called cilia line these airways and clear out dust and pollen. This system handles daily exposure well but struggles if you smoke. These airways connect to about 600 million tiny air sacs where oxygen enters your blood.

When lung cancer develops, cells grow wildly and harm this system, causing about 220,000 new cases and 125,000 deaths each year in the U.S. (American Cancer Society, 2025a). The good news? AI and other tools can help you prevent it, catch it early, and lower your risks.

## Smoking: The Leading Cause

Smoking causes 80–90% of lung cancer cases. This includes cigarettes, vaping devices, and marijuana. Cigarettes carry nicotine and harmful chemicals. Doctors measure exposure in pack-years: smoking one pack daily for 1 year. Marijuana gets counted in joint-years and can deliver twice the cancer-causing chemicals as tobacco. Marijuana smokers often breathe in deeply and hold smoke longer. This leaves more toxins in their lungs.

Many people view vaping as safer than smoking. This thinking is wrong and dangerous. Recent research shows people who both smoke and vape have four times higher lung cancer risk than those who only smoke cigarettes.

Vaping devices, like e-cigarettes, don't have tobacco, but they still make harmful chemicals, such as acrolein, formaldehyde, and metals like nickel and lead. These come from heating the liquid in vapes, which can cause health problems. We don't know for sure if vaping causes cancer because vaping is too new for long-term studies, but early research shows it can hurt your lungs by causing swelling and damage (Gotts et al., 2019). As a doctor, I've seen that chronic inflammation often precedes cancer, which makes these changes concerning.

Both vaping and smoking cigarettes damage the cilia. Vaping makes a wetter, liquid-like mist, while cigarette smoke is drier, but both can slow down or stop the cilia from working right (Chung et al., 2019). This makes it harder for your lungs to stay clean, letting harmful stuff stick around longer. Scientists aren't sure yet if vaping hurts cilia more than smoking, but both are bad for your lungs in different ways.

### Smoking and Lung Cancer in Different Communities

Different groups of people have different challenges when it comes to smoking and lung cancer. Understanding these differences helps create better programs to help people quit smoking.

White Americans have smoking rates of about 14% among adults. Their lung cancer rates match their smoking patterns and how easy it is for them to get healthcare (American Cancer Society, 2025b). White smokers often have better access to programs that help them quit smoking, though this depends a lot on how much money they have and where they live.

Black Americans face special challenges with smoking and lung cancer despite having similar smoking rates—also about 14%. There's an important difference in the type of cigarettes they smoke. A huge 85% of Black smokers use menthol cigarettes, compared to only 30% of White smokers (CDC, 2024b). Menthol cigarettes are particularly dangerous because the menthol cools your throat, making it easier to inhale deeper into your lungs. This deeper smoking may increase cancer risk and makes these cigarettes much harder to quit.

Black Americans also die from lung cancer more often than White Americans, even though they get lung cancer at similar rates. This happens mainly because it's harder for them to get early screening and treatment. Culturally tailored programs work much better for Black communities—the Pathways to Freedom video intervention, which draws on religion/spirituality, family, and community support, increased the odds of quitting by 50–60% compared to using quitline services alone (Webb Hooper et al., 2023). AI-powered versions of these culturally specific approaches could help even more people quit successfully.

Hispanic Americans have lower smoking rates at about 9.8%. But they face challenges like language barriers and cultural beliefs that make quitting harder—such as viewing smoking as a normal part of social life or stress relief (American Cancer Society, 2025b). Programs that involve the whole family work best in Hispanic communities. Spanish-language AI apps that understand cultural values and family relationships could help 25–30% more people quit successfully.

American Indian and Alaska Native people have the highest smoking rates of any racial/ethnic group at 27.1%, leading to very high lung cancer rates (CDC, 2024a). Traditional tobacco use for ceremonies makes quitting complicated. AI tools that understand the difference between ceremonial and everyday smoking, while respecting cultural practices, work best for these communities.

Asian Americans have among the lowest smoking rates at about 7.1%, though they face unique challenges including stigma around discussing smoking and significant variations across different Asian ethnic groups (Truth Initiative, 2020). Private AI quitting tools that let people participate without giving their names, while providing culturally sensitive education, could help more Asian communities get involved.

### Quitting Smoking: General Strategies and AI Support

Quitting smoking is the best step you can take for your health. Many tools can help, even if you've tried before. Most people need several attempts to quit for good. Each attempt teaches you about triggers. For example, you might crave a cigarette while out with friends who smoke at a bar at 10:30 PM much more than at 10:30 AM on Tuesday morning. Apps can spot these risky times.

### AI-Powered Apps for Smoking Cessation

Several apps have shown strong results in helping people quit smoking. While these apps are helpful tools, combining them with medical support gives you the best chance of success. These are current ones, but use: "What are the current AI-powered smoking cessation apps available, their key features, success rates, and costs?" to update the list and features.

- **QuitSure:** Uses mindfulness and therapy to reduce withdrawal symptoms. About 50% of users feel fewer symptoms. The app tracks smoking patterns to find high-risk times for alerts.
- **Smoke Free:** Provides coaching and community support. It helps 15–20% of users stay smoke-free for 6 months when used with other methods. Users can track cravings and get coping strategies.
- **QuitGenius:** Uses AI to analyze data from fitness trackers. It monitors things like heart rate patterns. Research shows it can increase quit rates by 36% compared to usual methods.
- **Kwit:** Tracks money saved, time since last cigarette, and cravings. It uses game features with milestones. Users log triggers tied to specific times or events.
- **quitSTART:** This free CDC app provides tips, challenges, and inspiration. It tracks cravings and offers games and coping tips during high-risk periods like weekend evenings.
- **EasyQuit:** Features tracking tools and gradual quitting options. It shows health improvement stats. While it has fewer real-time alerts than other apps, users rate it highly for ease of use.
- **CultureQuit:** Provides advice that fits your cultural background. Early research shows these approaches increase quit rates by 41% for Black smokers who use menthol cigarettes.
- **Community Health AI:** Connects users with online support groups. These groups understand your specific cultural background and smoking patterns.

Quitting smoking is absolutely possible, and you have proof all around you. More than 70 million Americans have successfully quit smoking, showing that freedom from cigarettes is achievable. While different methods work for different people, the winning formula comes down to determination and persistence. Most long-term quitters made an average of six to seven attempts before succeeding permanently. This doesn't mean relapse is necessary—some people quit on their first try. But if you've tried before and weren't successful, you're not alone, and each attempt brings you closer to success.

The key is learning from each attempt. Every time you quit, even briefly, you're training your brain and body to live without cigarettes. You're identifying your triggers, testing different strategies, and building the skills you'll need for permanent success. Think of previous attempts not as failures but as practice runs that make your next attempt stronger.

The best results come from using medicine and counseling together, but many people successfully quit on their own too. For those ready to work with their doctor, varenicline (Chantix/Champix) plus counseling works best—about 25–30% of people quit for at least 6 months (Cahill et al., 2016). Nicotine patches or gum plus counseling is nearly as good, helping 20–25% of people quit.

For the do-it-yourselfers, nicotine replacement products from the drugstore can really help. Using patches or gum on your own gives you about a 10–15% chance of quitting—much better than the 3–5% who succeed with cold turkey. The key is finding what works for you and not giving up if the first method doesn't stick.

What works best is different for each person. It depends on how long you've smoked, how many times you've tried to quit, and what you prefer. If you've tried to quit several times before, using both a nicotine patch AND gum or lozenges works better than using just one. This combo can boost your chances by 15–35% more than using one product alone (Lindson et al., 2019). Talk to your doctor to find the best mix of medicine and support for you.

### Lung Cancer Among Nonsmokers: Radon as the Leading Cause

For people who don't smoke, other factors become more important. Radon gas is the biggest cause of lung cancer in nonsmokers, causing about 21,000 deaths yearly in the U.S.—that's about half as many as die in car crashes each year (Environmental Protection Agency, 2023). This radioactive gas has no color, odor, or taste. It's truly a silent danger. Radon exists in all 50 states, but places like Alaska, South Dakota, and Pennsylvania often have higher levels.

Every home should be tested at least once. Radon levels can vary a lot even between neighboring houses. High-rise apartments above the third floor have lower risk. This is because radon mostly comes from soil. But it can still enter through concrete or water. If a test shows levels at or above 4 picocuries per liter, hire a certified professional. They can install a system like vent pipes with fans. These pull radon from beneath your home. Sealing cracks and adding ventilation also helps. These repairs cost about $700–1,500, but they're well worth it to make your home safe—just test again afterward to be sure.

Simple test kits that cost $10–20 can detect radon in your home. For ongoing monitoring, smart devices like AirThings Wave continuously track radon levels and send alerts to your phone when levels get too high. These devices connect to air quality apps that help you keep your home safe by showing you radon trends over time.

Air pollution from cars, factories, and wildfire smoke also raises your lung cancer risk. Tiny particles in dirty air can damage lung cells over time, especially during outdoor exercise when you breathe harder and deeper.

Smart air quality apps like AirNow, PurpleAir, and Breezometer use AI to predict tomorrow's air quality in your area. On high pollution days, these apps might suggest working out indoors instead of jogging outside. Some send morning alerts telling you the best times for outdoor exercise—usually early morning before trafic picks up.

During wildfire season, these tools become really valuable. When smoke makes the sky look orange and you can smell it in the air, that's when you actually need to stay inside. The same goes for those really smoggy summer days in big cities when you can see the haze. Most of the time, though, the air is fine for your regular activities. These apps help you know the difference between truly dangerous days and normal city air.

## Screening for Early Lung Cancer Detection

Finding lung cancer early greatly improves survival rates and treatment outcomes. Low-dose CT scans are the best screening tool available. These scans use 90% less radiation than standard CT scans and provide detailed images of lung tissue.

Medical groups recommend these scans for current or former smokers between ages 50 and 80 who have at least a 20 pack-year smoking history—that's like smoking a pack a day for 20 years or 2 packs a day for 10 years. If you smoked less than this, like just during college or your twenties, you typically don't qualify for screening under current guidelines.

But here's what's important: if you're worried about your lung cancer risk for any reason—family history, radon exposure, or even lighter smoking—talk to your doctor. Some doctors will order the scan anyway if you're anxious about it and willing to pay out of pocket (usually $200–400). The peace of mind might be worth it. You can also ask an AI assistant about screening guidelines for your specific smoking history, then discuss this information with your doctor.

Research shows that these scans reduce lung cancer deaths by 20% compared to regular chest X-rays, which often miss small tumors in the early stages when they're easiest to treat. There's also good news for people who can't get CT scans or need quick screening: AI programs are now making regular X-rays better at finding lung problems. These AI helpers can detect lung nodules that doctors might miss (Nam et al., 2019). In one study, doctors found lung problems about 65% of the time on their own. But with AI help, they found them 70% of the time. The AI also helped them avoid false alarms (Sim et al., 2020). These programs help doctors spot tiny spots that human eyes might miss. Finding these spots early means cancer can be treated when it's still small. The good news is that Medicare and most health insurance plans will pay for low-dose CT scans if you're at high risk for lung cancer.

### Action Steps and Privacy Considerations

When using AI apps for lung health monitoring, protecting your personal information is important. While lung scan results and health history are sensitive, any genetic data these apps collect requires extra care since it's permanent and affects your family too. Choose apps that comply with health privacy regulations. Review their data-sharing policies carefully. Pick apps that store sensitive information directly on your device rather than uploading it to cloud servers. Your smoking patterns or home air quality data can improve your health outcomes. But this information should remain under your control.

## Looking Forward

The future of lung health looks dramatically different from the smoking-dominated landscape of the past. We're entering an era where lung cancer becomes increasingly preventable, and when it does occur, it's caught early enough to treat successfully.

AI is transforming lung cancer prevention in ways that address both traditional and emerging threats. Smart home systems will continuously monitor radon levels and air quality, automatically adjusting ventilation when needed. Your phone will track local pollution levels and suggest the safest times for outdoor exercise. For people trying to quit smoking, AI apps will become incredibly sophisticated, predicting your craving patterns and intervening with personalized strategies before you reach for a cigarette.

Screening is becoming more precise and accessible. AI-enhanced CT scans can now detect lung cancers when they're still tiny and highly treatable. Soon, breath tests may identify cancer markers years before tumors become visible on scans. These tests could be as simple as breathing into a device at your doctor's office or even at home.

Getting ready for this AI-powered approach means staying curious about new capabilities and keeping your health information organized. But here's the bottom line: AI is becoming an incredibly sophisticated health assistant, but it's just that—an assistant. Your healthcare team is still essential for diagnosis, treatment decisions, and serious medical concerns.

The goal isn't just preventing lung cancer—it's helping everyone breathe easier and live healthier lives. AI is making this possible by turning complex environmental and medical data into simple, daily actions that protect your lungs for life.

CHAPTER 10

# BREATHING ROOM: AI'S BOOST FOR YOUR LUNGS

Your lungs are unsung heroes, quietly handling about 2,100–2,400 gallons of air every day—enough to fill a small truck. They sift through billions of tiny particles, from dust to pollen, with a clever system of hair-like cilia sweeping out intruders and immune cells neutralizing threats. Most of us breathe without a second thought, but for millions, conditions like asthma, chronic obstructive pulmonary disease (COPD), and other respiratory challenges make every breath a conscious effort. This is where AI comes in—not as a cure but as a partner to help you understand, manage, and possibly prevent these issues. This chapter explores how AI can empower you to take charge of your respiratory health, whether you're dealing with wheezing or shortness of breath or simply want to keep your lungs in top shape.

## Understanding Your Lungs with AI

Think of your lungs as a filter and a pump rolled into one. They're tough but not invincible. Asthma tightens the airways.

COPD damages the tiny air sacs. A clogged nose or throat can throw things off too.

AI helps by finding patterns in your data. If you've got a smartwatch or fitness tracker, it's already tracking your heart rate and sleep. Many newer models also track oxygen levels. Add an AI app, and it can spot patterns like changes in your breathing rate during sleep or dips in oxygen levels that hint at trouble. You don't need to be a doctor to use this. AI keeps it simple and alerts you when something is worth checking with a professional.

### Asthma: Managing the Squeeze

Asthma makes the tubes in your lungs get tight and swollen. Things like dust, pollen, cold air, or exercise can trigger an asthma attack. When this happens, breathing feels like trying to suck air through a straw—it's hard and makes you tired. Millions of Americans have asthma, but the good news is that AI technology can help you manage it better. Apps like Propeller keep track of your breathing and check the air quality where you are. These apps can warn you when the air might trigger your asthma. If you're wheezing more than normal, the AI tracks it along with your other symptoms. Then it can tell you when to use your inhaler or when you should call your doctor.

Pulmonary function tests (PFTs)—you blow into a machine to measure lung capacity—are the gold standard for diagnosis. AI can't run the test, but it can remind you to schedule one and help you understand the results—like if your airflow is restricted more than normal.

### COPD: Tackling the Long Haul

COPD is a slow burn, often tied to smoking but not always. It's actually a group of lung diseases, with emphysema and chronic bronchitis being the most common types. In emphysema, the tiny air sacs in your lungs get damaged, making it hard to exhale fully. Think of it as a balloon that won't deflate properly. Chronic bronchitis causes the airways to become inflamed and produce too much mucus, making you cough constantly. Many people have both conditions at the same time.

More than 16 million people in the U.S. have been diagnosed with COPD, though millions more likely have it without knowing (CDC, 2023). Smoking is the biggest culprit—past or present, it accounts for most cases. However, other risks, like air pollution or a rare genetic condition called alpha-1 antitrypsin deficiency, can also play a role.

AI helps by monitoring your oxygen levels through a pulse oximeter (a little clip on your finger) and flagging when they drop too low. It can also track your activity—say, if climbing stairs gets harder—and nudge you toward a PFT. If it's below normal, COPD might be the reason. Here, AI keeps you proactive, not panicked.

### Alpha-1 Antitrypsin Deficiency: The Hidden Factor

About 1 in 2,500 people have severe alpha-1 antitrypsin (AAT) deficiency with two copies of the defective gene. Your lungs face irritants constantly—dust, pollution, smoke. Your body fights back with inflammation, which is helpful at first. But inflammation needs to be turned off after it's done its job, before it becomes chronic and starts damaging lung tissue.

That's where AAT comes in. Your liver makes this protein to calm the inflammation down after it has protected your lungs but before it can hurt you. With severe AAT deficiency, you don't make enough of it. The inflammation keeps going, breaking down lung tissue. Add smoking, and the damage speeds up fast—causing emphysema decades earlier than normal.

But there's more to this story. About 1 in 40 people carry one normal gene and one defective gene—they're called MZ carriers. That's more common than peanut allergies and about the same chance as having twins. I'm one of them. These carriers make about half the normal amount of AAT. If they don't smoke and avoid heavy lung irritants, most stay healthy. But smoking or working in jobs with constant dust, chemical, or smoke exposure can trigger early lung disease in carriers too.

I didn't know about my carrier status until I worked at the Mayo Clinic. After a cold or the flu, I would get a cough that lingered 2–3 weeks—I sounded terrible and the coughing was exhausting. That's when I got tested and learned I was a carrier. I'm sharing my story because I want you to get the same great medical care I've had.

This is where AI becomes your early warning system. AI apps that track lung function patterns might spot trouble before you feel sick—catching unusually fast decline in breathing capacity or oxygen levels, especially if you're young and otherwise healthy. These red flags could prompt your doctor to test for AAT deficiency, which often goes undiagnosed for years.

AI can't fix your genes, but it can help you manage the risk. If you've got a family history or early breathing trouble, AI can prompt you to get a blood test to check your alpha-1 levels. Genetic testing, covered in Chapter 3, shows if you're at risk. AI can then remind you to avoid smoke, monitor your symptoms, and push for regular PFTs to catch changes early. AI platforms can also combine your genetic information with lifestyle data to create personalized risk profiles, helping you and your doctor decide if yearly screening makes sense. This is especially valuable for firefighters, construction workers, welders, and others with heavy occupational exposures. If you're a carrier in one of these jobs, avoiding smoking and reducing lung irritant exposure isn't just good advice—it's critical protection for your lungs.

### Clearing the Upper Airway

Breathing issues can come from a blocked nose or throat, like from allergies. This may cause snoring or feeling stuffed up all day. Apps like Sleep Cycle track irregular breathing at night, as described in Chapter 6. Smart humidifiers with AI adjust room air to ease congestion. If it's serious, see a doctor, but AI offers daily clues, like low sleep scores on high-pollen days.

### Taking Action: Your Next Steps with AI

Want better breathing? Try Propeller or AirNow to track asthma or air quality. Use these apps with local air data to log symptoms like wheezing for asthma or breathlessness for COPD. Test your home for mold with kits ($10–20). If alpha-1 runs in your family, ask about genetic testing. Share AI insights with your doctor to stay proactive.

### Looking Forward

The future of breathing health is exciting, and it's happening right now. Smart inhalers can already track when you use your medication and warn you days before an asthma attack might happen. They notice tiny changes in your breathing that you can't even feel yet. Soon, these inhalers will connect to local weather apps to warn you when pollen or pollution levels are dangerous in your area.

For people with COPD, new tools will make daily life much easier. Small wearable patches will check your oxygen levels all day without you feeling them. Your home's air filtration system will automatically clean the air better when it senses you're having breathing trouble. These aren't science fiction—companies are testing them in real hospitals today.

AI will also help people with genetic lung conditions like alpha-1 antitrypsin deficiency. Instead of just telling you that you're at risk, AI will create a personal protection plan for your whole life. It might suggest safe jobs that avoid dust and smoke or design exercise routines that make your lungs stronger.

The best part? These tools will work on your regular smartphone, no matter where you live. Someone in a small town will get the same quality help as someone in a big city. The technology isn't replacing doctors—it's like having a smart assistant that watches for trouble and gets help before you get really sick.

The goals are simple: to help you breathe easier and without worry. All these new tools—from smart inhalers to genetic tests—have one job: to make managing lung problems so easy that breathing stays as natural as it should be.

CHAPTER 11

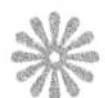

# INFECTIOUS DISEASES AND AI: STAYING AHEAD OF HIDDEN THREATS

Getting sick is never fun, but what if you could stop illness before it starts? Or know exactly what to do when symptoms hit? AI tools can help you stay one step ahead of infections like flu, COVID-19, and Lyme disease. Think of AI as your personal health coach—always ready with smart advice based on the latest medical knowledge. This chapter shows how AI helps prevent illness and manage symptoms with simple questions.

## Prevention: Building Your Shield Before You Get Sick

The best way to handle infections is to avoid them entirely. AI excels at helping you track important protections like vaccines and warning you about disease outbreaks or health risks in your area. Think of prevention as building layers of protection—vaccines, awareness of local threats, and smart daily habits.

Vaccines are your strongest shield against many diseases, but tracking what you need can be confusing. When did you last get a tetanus shot? Are you protected against measles? AI can help sort this out. Start by gathering your vaccine records from your doctor's office or pharmacy.

Ada Health is a medical AI app that acts like a symptom checker and health guide. Ask Ada Health: "I'm [your age], in [your city]. Which vaccines do I need?" The AI will check current guidelines and tell you what's missing. For example, if you're over 50, you might need a shingles vaccine. If you're planning to travel, you might need protection against diseases common in other countries. The AI can also explain how well vaccines work—like how the measles vaccine prevents illness in 97 out of 100 people who get both recommended doses.

Tom, 30, got a measles booster after AI warned of local cases. Measles deserves special attention because it spreads incredibly easily through the air when someone coughs or sneezes. One infected person can spread measles to 12–18 others in a crowded room. If you weren't vaccinated as a child or only got one dose, AI might suggest getting a booster. This is especially important if you live in an area with low vaccination rates or plan to travel.

AI can send you alerts when serious diseases break out in your area. Apps like HealthMap and the CDC's Alert system only message you when there's a real health threat that might change your plans. For example, they'll warn you about measles at your child's school or unusual flu spreading in your zip code. These warnings come from real lab tests.

The best part? You don't have to check every day. The apps only alert you when you need to do something. You might get messages like: "Strep throat is spreading in your area—watch for sore throats in kids" or "COVID cases went up 40% near you—think about skipping indoor crowds or wearing a mask at concerts and basketball games this week."

### Treatment: Smart Decisions When Illness Strikes

Carmen, 45, used AI to check her fever and avoid an ER visit. Even with the best prevention, sometimes you get sick. AI can help you figure out if it's just a cold or something that needs medical attention. It can also guide you toward safe treatments and help you know when to seek professional care. The goal isn't to replace your doctor but to help you make smart decisions about when and how to get help.

When you're feeling awful, AI can help check your symptoms and guide you toward the right care, whether at home or while traveling. Ask Ada Health: "I have fever and cough. Is it a cold or serious?" The AI will compare your symptoms to patterns of different illnesses and warn you about serious signs like fever over 102°F, trouble breathing, severe headache, or chest pain that need quick medical attention.

When your symptoms change or you're away from home, you can update the AI to help decide if you need urgent care, emergency services, or home treatment. However, always trust your gut—get medical help (call your doctor, go to urgent care, or go to the emergency room) if you feel seriously ill, even if AI says to wait.

Before reaching for over-the-counter medicines, AI can make sure they're safe with any medications you already take. Some drugs, like blood thinners, can mix badly with over-the-counter medicines. Ask: "I take apixaban for blood clots and have a headache and fever. What over-the-counter medicines are safe for me? Are there any dangerous combinations I should avoid?" In this case, the AI might warn against ibuprofen, which can increase bleeding risk when combined with these medications and suggest acetaminophen instead. This simple check can prevent serious complications.

Getting sick away from home presents special challenges, but the same AI symptom assessment can help you find appropriate local care quickly. Ask your AI: "I'm in [specific location] and have these symptoms: [list them]. Find local urgent care centers, emergency rooms, or walk-in clinics near me. Based on my symptoms, what type of care do I need?" The AI can locate nearby medical facilities, provide addresses and phone numbers, and help you decide whether your symptoms need urgent care or emergency care.

### Tick Bites: A Special Case

Found a tick? This is where AI really shines with step-by-step guidance. Ask WebMD's AI or another health AI for removal steps and Lyme risk assessment. AI will walk you through using fine-tipped tweezers to pull straight out without twisting, storing the tick in a sealed bag with a damp paper towel, and finding local labs that test ticks for Lyme disease.

It can tell you if your area has high Lyme disease risk—in some places, half of all ticks carry the Lyme bacteria—and what symptoms to watch for over the next 3–30 days. Testing the tick can help your doctor make better treatment decisions: if it's negative, you might avoid unnecessary antibiotics that could trigger allergies or upset your gut bacteria, and if it's positive, you're more likely to get the antibiotics you need to prevent serious long-term problems. With about 476,000 people getting Lyme disease each year in the U.S., this guidance really matters (Kugeler et al., 2021).

For other concerns, like wondering if zinc lozenges or vitamin C will help your cold, AI can check the latest research and tell you what's worth trying and what might interact with your current medications, including those blood thinners that affect so many treatment choices.

Getting ready for this AI-powered approach means staying curious about new tools and keeping your health information organized. Start building comfort with asking detailed health questions now. But here's the bottom line: AI is becoming an incredibly sophisticated health assistant, but it's just that—an assistant. Your healthcare team is still essential for diagnosis, treatment decisions, and serious medical concerns. Most importantly, remember that even the most advanced AI works best when combined with regular medical care—it's becoming an incredibly sophisticated assistant, but your healthcare team remains essential for serious medical decisions.

## Looking Forward

Infectious disease prevention is entering an era of real-time intelligence that will transform how we protect ourselves and our communities. We're moving from reacting to outbreaks after they spread to predicting and preventing them before they take hold.

AI systems are being developed that will track your infection risk based on where you are, what you do, and your health. In the future, symptom checking will be much smarter. AI will look at more than just the symptoms you report. It will also notice small changes in your voice, how you type, or data from fitness trackers. This helps find illness before you even feel sick. Catching illness early means you can take action or get treatment when it works best.

What gives me the most hope is how AI will democratize access to high-quality medical guidance. Whether you're in a major city or a remote rural area, you'll have access to the same level of intelligent symptom assessment and treatment recommendations. This could be life-changing for people who live far from medical facilities or have limited access to healthcare.

Keeping track of vaccines and disease outbreaks can be complicated. AI tools can help by organizing your vaccine records and alerting you to relevant health risks in your area—but only if you choose to use them. You'll get personalized reminders about vaccines and health alerts based on your schedule and situation, not one-size-fits-all warnings. You control what information you share and what alerts you receive. The goal is a personal health assistant who keeps you informed without overwhelming you, so you can make the best decisions for your family.

The goal isn't to make you worry more about getting sick—it's to help you worry less by giving you the tools and knowledge to stay healthy. AI is creating a world where infectious diseases become manageable challenges rather than unpredictable threats, keeping you and your loved ones safer through intelligent, personalized protection.

# PART 3

# Personalized Prevention: AI Tools for Proactive Health Management

CHAPTER 12

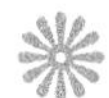

# YOUR AI MEDICATION ASSISTANT: ANOTHER LAYER OF PROTECTION

Juggling multiple medications is something many of us face every day. Whether it's prescriptions from different doctors, over-the-counter medicines, or daily supplements, keeping track of everything can feel overwhelming. While our healthcare system has several safety measures in place, adding your own check with AI tools gives you an extra layer of protection and puts you in greater control of your health.

## The Safety Net That Sometimes Has Holes

Your healthcare system already works hard to keep you safe with three main protective measures. Your doctor reviews your existing medications and allergies when prescribing something new. Electronic medical records can automatically flag potential medication problems. And your pharmacy reviews your prescriptions for conflicts with other medications you're taking.

Healthcare systems face big problems with medication safety when patients see many doctors. Studies show that about 26–44% of patients have medication errors when they move between different care settings (Bonaudo et al., 2018). Doctors struggle to track medicines given by other specialists. The problem gets worse when hospitals and clinics can't share patient records (Heyworth et al., 2013).

Studies show that medication errors happen more often when there's no formal system to check medicines. Poor communication between doctors also causes these mix-ups (Barnsteiner, 2008). These errors happen for common reasons. Your doctors don't talk to each other. You use different pharmacies. Or you forget to tell doctors about all your medicines.

### How AI Can Help You Check Your Medications

Think of AI as your additional health advocate who's available whenever you need guidance. Using AI to check your medications is straightforward and can provide insights your healthcare team might miss.

First, make a complete list of everything you take—prescriptions, over-the-counter medicines, and supplements. For each one, include the name, strength (milligrams), how you take it, how often, and when. Don't forget to add your medication allergies and what reactions you've experienced. Keep this list updated whenever changes occur, as you'll use it regularly with both your healthcare provider and AI tools.

Once you have this information, you can use AI tools to analyze it. Several options are available in 2025, including LLMs like Claude (by Anthropic), ChatGPT (by OpenAI), Grok (by xAI), and Gemini (by Google). There are also medication-specific apps such as MedWise, which provides medication risk scores; Epocrates, which includes a drug interaction checker; and Medisafe, a medication management tool with interaction alerts.

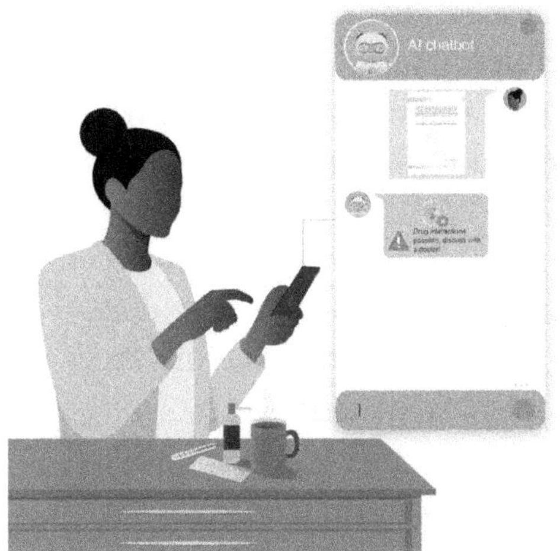

AI apps can help check drug interactions and pharmacogenomic compatibility

When using these tools, be specific with your request. Here's a prompt you can copy and use with any AI assistant:

> I'd like to check my medications for potential problems. Here's my complete list, including prescriptions, over-the-counter medicines, and supplements. For each, I've included the name, strength, and how I take it. I've also listed my medication allergies. Could you please check for any interactions between these medications, suggest the best times to take each one (morning/evening, with/without food), identify any vitamins or minerals these medications might drain from my body, and recommend any monitoring or supplements I should discuss with my doctor?

## Beyond Interactions: What AI Can Tell You

AI can help identify much more than just drug interactions. Many medications can drain important vitamins and minerals from your body—something rarely discussed during doctor visits. For example, statin medications drain coenzyme Q10, which helps your cells produce energy. Acid reducers can lower vitamin B12, magnesium, and calcium levels over time.

Let me show you what this looks like in practice. Here's an actual conversation with Claude AI:

> Charlie asked: "This is a list of my medicines and my allergies to medicines. Are there any that interact with each other? Any special instructions—morning or evening? Full stomach or empty? List the supplements that these medications drain and any suggestions for taking supplements to keep this from happening.

Medications:

- Lisinopril 20 mg once daily
- Atorvastatin 40 mg once daily
- Metformin 500 mg twice daily
- Aspirin 81 mg once daily
- Levothyroxine 50 mcg once daily
- Vitamin D3 1,000 IU daily
- Calcium 500 mg daily

Allergies:

- Penicillin (rash)
- Sulfa drugs (difficulty breathing)"

Claude responded with several important observations: First, it noted that calcium supplements can reduce levothyroxine absorption, making it less effective, and recommended taking these at least 4 hours apart. It also mentioned that taking aspirin and lisinopril together may slightly reduce the blood pressure-lowering effect of lisinopril, though this is usually managed with monitoring.

For timing recommendations, Claude explained that levothyroxine works best when taken first thing in the morning on an empty stomach, at least 30–60 minutes before other medications or food. It noted that atorvastatin is more effective when taken in the evening, as most cholesterol is produced overnight. The AI recommended taking metformin with meals to reduce stomach upset and aspirin in the morning with food to reduce stomach irritation.

Regarding nutrient losses, Claude pointed out that atorvastatin drains CoQ10, which may contribute to muscle pain, and suggested considering a CoQ10 supplement (100–200 mg daily). AI correctly identifies that your statin might be causing muscle pain and suggests CoQ10, that's helpful—but incomplete. Here's what your doctor needs to check: Are your muscle enzymes elevated? (A blood test tells us if there's actual muscle damage.) Would switching to a different statin work better for your body? Some people do great on rosuvastatin but terrible on atorvastatin. Most importantly—do you actually need the statin at all? I've had patients where rechecking their cardiac risk showed they could safely stop the medication entirely. One patient's muscle pain turned out to be from low thyroid, not the statin at all. Your doctor can sort through these possibilities; AI is just making educated guesses.

It also noted that metformin can lower vitamin B12 and folate levels over time, making a B-complex supplement potentially beneficial. Finally, it mentioned that lisinopril may drain zinc and suggested considering a zinc supplement (15–30 mg daily).

This example shows how much valuable information you can get with a single question to an AI assistant. Notice how Claude identified a potential interaction between calcium and levothyroxine that might be overlooked and provided specific timing recommendations to avoid the problem.

### Personalized Medicine: Understanding the Uniqueness of Your Body

We all process medications differently. Have you ever noticed that some medicines affect you more strongly than others? This isn't just your imagination—it's biology at work. Your liver breaks down medications using special proteins called enzymes, particularly through a pathway called cytochrome P450 that handles 70–80% of drugs. This process is called metabolism or detoxification. It's the same system that sobers you up after drinking alcohol, which is why you need to take most medications daily or more often—your body is constantly breaking them down.

Here's where it gets personal: people have enzymes that work at different speeds—some are fast, some are slow, and most fall somewhere in between. If you have fast enzymes for a particular drug, you might need higher doses because your body clears it quickly. If you have slow enzymes, you might need lower doses to avoid side effects. Here's the tricky part: different medications use different enzymes, so you could be a fast metabolizer for one drug and a slow metabolizer for another.

If you're interested in understanding your unique medication processing, genetic testing (pharmacogenomics) is now available. Some tests require your doctor to order them, while others can be ordered directly by consumers. The cost varies widely, from $250 to $1,000 or more, depending on how many genes are tested and your insurance coverage. Many insurance plans cover these tests when deemed medically necessary, though coverage is not guaranteed. Sample collection is simple and noninvasive, typically involving either a blood draw or cheek swab, with the latter being the most common method due to its convenience. You can also ask AI: "What pharmacogenomic tests are available, and what do they typically cost?"

This test examines your genes related to drug processing and can help predict how you'll respond to certain medications. The results can be particularly helpful when combined with AI analysis of your medication regimen.

## Working With Your Healthcare Team

Using AI does not mean replacing your healthcare providers. It means partnering with them for better care. By identifying potential issues before they become problems, you can have more informed conversations with your doctor.

When you discover something through your AI consultation, bring it up at your next appointment: "I was reading about statins draining CoQ10. Is that something I should be concerned about?" This approach shows you're engaged in your health and opens the door for productive discussions.

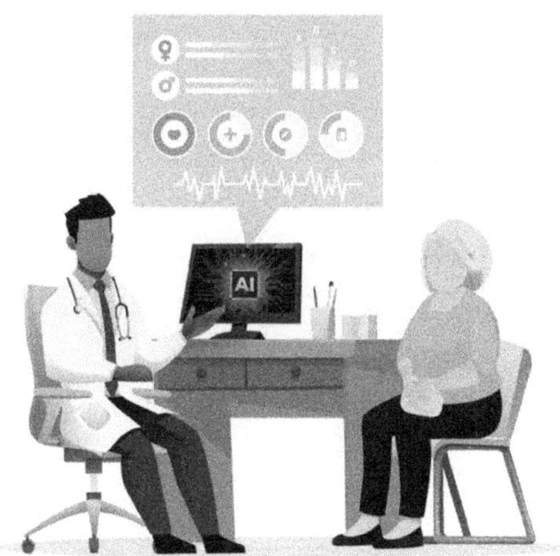


AI tools can support medical expertise and enhance doctor-patient communication

By combining the expertise of healthcare professionals with AI technology, you're creating a stronger safety net for your health.

## Staying Up to Date with AI Medication Safety

Since technology evolves rapidly, you'll want to check for advances in this field periodically. Here are some prompts you can use with any AI assistant to find the latest developments:

You might ask: "What are the newest AI tools for medication safety and interaction checking developed in the past year?" This will help you discover both consumer apps and professional systems that have recently emerged.

To stay informed about research in this area, try asking: "Have there been any major studies or clinical trials on the effectiveness of AI for medication management published in the last 2 years?"

If you're already using a specific app, you can ask: "What new features have been added to [name of app you use] for medication safety." This will help you take advantage of any updates or improvements.

Finally, to ensure you're aware of any limitations or concerns, you might ask: "Are there any new concerns or limitations about using AI for medication checking that healthcare professionals are discussing?"

These questions will help you discover new tools and understand how the field is evolving, ensuring you always have access to the most helpful resources for managing your medications safely.

CHAPTER 13

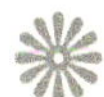

# SUPPLEMENTS AND AI: A SMART PATH TO BETTER HEALTH

Supplements are everywhere these days, and it's no wonder why. People are drawn to the idea of a quick boost for their health—something to fill in the gaps when life gets busy or diets fall short. With at least 30,000 different supplements available, from vitamins to herbs to fancy compounds promising antiaging miracles, the options can feel overwhelming. But here's the good news: you don't have to navigate this maze alone. With AI and some practical habits, you can make smarter choices about supplements and feel more confident about what you're putting into your body.

## The Vitamin Mystique: Why More Usually Isn't Better

The hype around vitamins comes from their dramatic power to cure deficiencies—and those stories are real. In the 1700s, sailors developed scurvy, a devastating disease that caused bleeding gums, tooth loss, and eventually death. The cure? Citrus fruits packed with vitamin C. Within days, dying sailors would recover. It seemed like magic.

Fast-forward to the early 1900s, when children with rickets—a bone disease that caused severe deformities—were cured with vitamin D from cod liver oil. Their twisted bones straightened, and they could walk again.

Consider vitamin A deficiency, a leading cause of preventable blindness in developing countries. My former Johns Hopkins dean, Alfred Sommer, achieved something remarkable by proving that simple vitamin A supplementation could prevent childhood blindness and death. His work has brought life and sight to millions of children worldwide—a truly life-changing intervention by a great man.

These miraculous recoveries created what I call the "vitamin mystique"—the belief that if vitamins can work such wonders for deficiencies, taking more must be even better. But here's the reality: when you're not deficient, vitamins and supplements provide mild benefits at best. Your body uses what it needs and either stores or flushes out the rest.

In fact, too much of even a good thing can become harmful. A 16th-century physician named Paracelsus said it best: "The dose makes the poison." Even water can hurt you if you drink too much—it can dilute the sodium in your blood to dangerous levels. The same goes for vitamins. Extra vitamin C won't prevent colds or give you super immunity; studies show it might shorten a cold by about a day, but most of it just ends up in your urine.

Focus on the most important vitamins and other supplements—like vitamin D and the B vitamins discussed below—that can actually be measured through blood tests. There are other vitamins and minerals that can be tested too, so talk to your doctor about checking your levels and supplementing based on what you need, not on marketing hype. If you're taking a handful or more of supplements each day, you're probably taking too many.

## New to Supplements? Start Here

If you're just getting started with supplements, don't worry—you don't need to become an expert overnight. The best first step is simple: ask your doctor for a vitamin D test at your next visit. For most people, vitamin D is the single most important vitamin or supplement to get right. This test is usually covered by insurance and gives you a clear picture of whether you need it. From there, you can build your knowledge gradually.

Here's something many people don't know: even safe supplements can cause problems if you take too much. For example, vitamin C doses above 2,000 mg per day can lead to crystal formation in your kidneys, potentially causing kidney stones. Research shows this risk is especially high in people already prone to kidney stones.

Remember, the FDA doesn't preapprove supplements as they do medications, so quality varies widely—sometimes dramatically. Here's what you need to know about supplement risks:

### Quality Control Issues

- Some supplements contain less (or more) of the active ingredient than listed on the label
- Contamination with heavy metals, bacteria, or other drugs has been found in various products
- Manufacturing standards vary significantly between companies

### What to Look For

- Third-party testing by NSF International, USP (United States Pharmacopeia), or ConsumerLab

- GMP (good manufacturing practices) certification
- Avoid products with unrealistic claims or those sold only online without company contact information
- Read labels for fillers like artificial colors—simpler ingredients are often better

Maria, a 38-year-old nurse, learned this lesson the hard way. "I bought a cheap magnesium supplement online that was giving me stomach problems. When I switched to a USP-verified brand, the problems disappeared. Turns out the cheap one had poor quality control and inconsistent dosing—some pills had twice the amount listed on the label."

### Understanding the Supplement Landscape

These supplements range from well-known vitamins to obscure products like milk thistle, horny goat weed, or shark cartilage that have little proven benefit. That's a lot to sort through! Some of these, like vitamin D and B vitamins, have solid science backing them and can make a real difference if your levels are low. Others have shakier evidence, and it's hard to know if they're helping or sitting in your system doing nothing—or worse.

Rachel, a 42-year-old software developer, knows this challenge all too well. "I used to have a bathroom drawer full of supplements—about 15 different bottles. I was spending nearly $200 a month but had no idea if they were actually doing anything," she explains. "Then I started tracking them with an AI app that analyzed my symptoms and lab tests alongside what I was taking. Turns out, only three of those supplements were making a measurable difference to my health."

## The Smart Approach: Focus on What You Can Measure

Here's a simple rule I follow: If you can't measure it, you probably don't need it. Out of all these thousands of options, only about 20 have reliable blood tests to check their levels in your body. That's less than 0.001% of all available supplements! The rest can't be measured directly, making it hard to know if they're working.

Take milk thistle, for example. It's popular for liver health, but there's no "milk thistle level" you can check. Without that, how do you know if you need more, or if you've already had too much? This is where focusing on measurable supplements makes sense.

## The 20 Supplements You Can Actually Test

| Supplement | What It Does | How It's Tested |
|---|---|---|
| Vitamin D | Bone health, immune function, mood | 25-hydroxyvitamin D blood test |
| Vitamin B12 | Brain function, energy, nerve health | B12 blood test |
| Iron | Oxygen transport, energy | Ferritin and transferrin tests |
| Magnesium | Muscle function, heart rhythm, sleep | Magnesium blood test |
| Omega-3 fatty acids | Heart health, brain function, inflammation | EPA/DHA blood test |
| Vitamin B9 (folate) | Cell division, DNA repair | Folate blood test |
| Zinc | Immune function, wound healing | Zinc blood test |
| Vitamin C | Immune function, collagen production | Ascorbic acid blood test |

| Supplement | What It Does | How It's Tested |
|---|---|---|
| Calcium | Bone health, muscle function | Calcium blood test |
| Selenium | Antioxidant protection, thyroid function | Selenium blood test |
| Vitamin A | Vision, immune function, cell growth | Retinol blood test |
| Vitamin E | Antioxidant protection, skin health | Tocopherol blood test |
| Vitamin K | Blood clotting, bone health | Vitamin K blood test |
| Copper | Iron absorption, connective tissue | Copper blood test |
| Iodine | Thyroid function, metabolism | Thyroid function tests |
| CoQ10 | Heart health, cellular energy<br>Taking a statin can lower your level | CoQ10 blood test |
| Vitamin B1 (thiamine) | Energy metabolism, nerve function | Thiamine blood test |
| Vitamin B2 (riboflavin) | Energy production, eye health | Riboflavin blood test |
| Vitamin B3 (niacin) | Cholesterol, brain function | Niacin blood test |
| Vitamin B6 (pyridoxine) | Brain development, immune function | Pyridoxine blood test |

## Key Supplements Worth Your Attention

Let's zoom in on the most important ones: vitamin D and B vitamins. Vitamin D keeps your bones strong, boosts your immune system, and may improve your mood.

Most medical organizations recommend vitamin D levels of at least 30 ng/mL for bone health. The Endocrine Society's 2011 guidelines suggested a preferred range of 40–60 ng/mL, noting that levels up to 100 ng/mL are safe (Holick et al., 2011). However, I aim for my patients to have levels around 70 ng/mL. This target is higher than current standard guidelines, but recent research suggests it may help protect against diseases like cancer and diabetes (Grant et al., 2025). The evidence for these extra benefits is still being studied, which is why most guidelines stick to lower targets focused mainly on bone health.

You may need 4,000–6,000 IU of vitamin D daily to reach 70 ng/mL, but always check with your doctor first to stay safe and avoid taking too much. Now, before you start taking 10,000 IU of vitamin D daily because AI calculated that's what you need to reach optimal levels, here's what happened to Jamail. He didn't tell me he was already taking calcium supplements for his bones plus a multivitamin with more calcium. Add high-dose vitamin D to that mix, and within 3 months he had painful kidney stones—his body absorbed too much calcium. Your doctor can check not just your vitamin D level but also your calcium and parathyroid hormone to make sure it's safe to supplement. We might also discover you're one of those people who need just 2,000 IU to maintain perfect levels, saving you money and avoiding problems.

### How AI Can Help

You can use AI tools, like free apps such as Cronometer or MyFitnessPal, to track your vitamin D intake from food and supplements. AI can also check your blood test results over time to see if your levels are improving or if you need to adjust your dose.

For example, you can ask an AI assistant: "I'm taking 5,000 IU of vitamin D daily and my last blood level was 50 ng/mL. Should I change my dose to reach 70 ng/mL?" AI can suggest questions to ask your doctor and keep you updated on new vitamin D research by searching for the latest studies. Just say: "Find me the newest research on vitamin D and health," and it can summarize findings in simple words to help you stay informed.

## B12: When "Normal" Isn't Optimal

Vitamin B12 is crucial for brain health and keeping homocysteine (a blood marker linked to heart and brain problems) in check. B12 deficiency is surprisingly common—affecting up to 6% of people over 70.

Here's the problem: The U.S. considers B12 levels above 200 pg/mL "normal," but Japan and parts of Europe use 500–550 pg/mL as their cutoff. Japan established this higher standard back in 1988, recognizing that lower levels might contribute to dementia (Mitsuyama & Kogoh, 1988). Interestingly, Japan has lower rates of Alzheimer's than the U.S., and while many factors contribute to this, their higher B12 standards might play a role.

Many experts warn about a "gray zone" between 200 and 500 pg/mL where people can have symptoms—memory problems, fatigue, nerve issues—even though their levels are considered normal (Pacholok & Stuart, 2011). More doctors now recognize that levels below 500 pg/mL may affect brain health.

The good news? B12 supplementation is extremely safe—your body simply flushes out what it doesn't need. I routinely recommend B12 to my patients, aiming for levels between 500–1,000 pg/mL. AI can help you track your B12 intake using apps like Cronometer and stay updated on the latest research. Always talk to your doctor about testing and supplementation.

Mark, a 58-year-old history teacher with persistent fatigue, tried multiple supplements without success. "My doctor ran tests but everything looked 'normal,' though at the low end," he shares. "I uploaded my results to an AI health platform that flagged borderline B12 and iron levels my doctor hadn't been concerned about. After 3 months of targeted supplementation, my energy improved dramatically, and follow-up tests showed I'd moved into the optimal range."

### B9 (Folate): More Than Just a Blood Vitamin

Folate (vitamin B9) is one of the most complex vitamins when it comes to brain health. It helps make neurotransmitters—the chemical messengers brain cells use to communicate, including serotonin, dopamine, and norepinephrine. Here's where it gets tricky: folate levels in your blood don't always reflect levels inside your cells or brain, where it actually does its work. To get folate into cells and across the blood-brain barrier, your body needs special receptors and transport proteins. That's where folinic acid comes in—a different form of B9 that can bypass these receptors and transport proteins to get directly into your cells and brain.

**Research shows that many children with autism—about 70%—have special antibodies that attack the folate receptor.** This protein helps carry folate (a key nutrient) into the brain. These antibodies can block folate from reaching the brain, even if blood tests show normal levels. This creates a shortage of folate in the brain, called cerebral folate deficiency, which can affect a child's development and behavior. (Frye et al., 2013; Rossignol & Frye, 2021)

Folinic acid (also called leucovorin) can get around these blocked pathways to deliver folate to the brain. That's why the FDA recently updated its use to treat cerebral folate deficiency in children showing autism symptoms. If your child has autism, don't start folinic acid on your own—but it's worth asking your pediatrician. They can test for these antibodies and see if folinic acid might help.

**For adults with chronic fatigue syndrome, early research suggests a significant number have experienced significant improvement with folinic acid treatment. Folinic acid is generally safe and available as an over-the-counter (OTC) supplement.** If AI symptom checkers or health apps suggest you might have CFS—or if you've been diagnosed—it's worth asking your doctor about trying folinic acid.

There's one more important piece: about 40% of people have a genetic variation (*MTHFR* mutation) that makes it harder to convert regular folic acid into its active form, methylfolate. You can determine if you have this through genetic testing, but many people simply take methylated B vitamins (like methylfolate and methylcobalamin) as insurance. If you don't need the methylated form, your body will just use it anyway without harm—but if you do need it, you'll get the B vitamins your body can actually use.

## Beyond Basic Vitamins: When Specialized Supplements Make Sense

Here's a myth we need to bust: the idea that supplements are always "safe" because they're natural.

That said, some supplements shine in specific situations. If you're on statins for cholesterol, they can lower CoQ10, which may cause muscle pain and fatigue. Adding a CoQ10 supplement might help restore your energy and support heart health. Omega-3 fatty acids are another good option—they're linked to less buildup in your arteries, and you can measure them in your blood.

Then there's berberine, which seems to help with insulin resistance—a common issue tied to prediabetes. A 2008 study found that berberine improved blood sugar control in patients with type 2 diabetes (Zhang et al., 2008). There are no direct blood tests for berberine, but the science is promising enough to discuss with your doctor.

## AI Tools: Free and Affordable Options

The good news is that many AI-powered supplement tools are free or low-cost, making them accessible to most people. Here are some options:

### Free Tools

- Cronometer (free version tracks nutrients from food and supplements)
- MyFitnessPal (basic nutrient tracking)
- Drug interaction checkers at Drugs.com let you check for potential problems between your medications and supplements. There are many cases of supplements interfering with prescription medicines—Always tell your physician what supplements you're taking, even if they don't ask.

### Low-Cost Options

- Cronometer Gold ($6/month for advanced features)
- MyTherapy (free with premium features available)
- InsideTracker (periodic promotions make it more affordable)

### For Those Without Tech Access

- Keep a written supplement and medication list
- Use basic blood tests covered by insurance
- Ask your pharmacist about drug interactions

Choose apps with strong privacy policies, and always confirm AI suggestions with your doctor to ensure accuracy.

AI supplement tracking platforms like Rootine and InsideTracker analyze your blood test results to identify deficiencies and track symptoms. They compare your supplement intake with your test results and adjust recommendations as new data come in. While some premium services can be expensive, many basic features are available at no cost.

### The Paper List: Your Most Important Tool

Surprisingly, here's the **most important takeaway about supplements** in this AI book in this high-tech era: **Keep a written list (in your wallet or purse) of everything you take—medications and supplements.** Carry it with you, update it when things change, and show it to your doctor at every visit. Why paper? Because most medical offices and emergency departments won't plug in a USB drive to read your list—they're worried about viruses and security risks. Cell phone reception in emergency departments is usually bad because of the leaded walls used for radiology protection. This list is a lifesaver, especially in an emergency.

Beyond this paper list, AI can take your supplement management to the next level. Apps can send reminders based on your routine, spot patterns in how supplements affect your symptoms, and check for dangerous combinations between your supplements and medications.

These interaction checks are crucial. A 2017 study found that many common supplements can either reduce how well your medications work or increase side effects (Asher et al., 2017). For example, St. John's wort can make birth control pills less effective, and fish oil can increase the effects of blood thinners.

Priya, a 63-year-old with several health conditions, takes seven prescription medications and four supplements. "I was worried about interactions," she says. "My cardiologist was concerned about my fish oil interfering with my blood thinner, but my rheumatologist recommended it for inflammation. I used an AI interaction checker that suggested taking the fish oil at a different time from my blood thinner. My next lab test showed each was working properly."

Bret, a 49-year-old with persistent brain fog, followed this strategy. "I was taking a multivitamin, fish oil, and vitamin D without much thought. After analyzing my blood work with an AI tool, I discovered I had borderline B12 levels and high inflammation markers. The AI suggested adding a specific form (methylated) of B12 and turmeric. Within 6 weeks, my focus improved dramatically, and my follow-up blood work showed my inflammation markers had dropped by 30%."

## Your Smart Supplement Strategy

Here's a simple approach to using AI for supplement optimization:

1. **Start with the basics.** Get blood tests for vitamin D and B12 through your doctor.
2. **Track your symptoms.** Note how you feel day to day using a free app or simple journal.

3. **Check for interactions.** Use free online tools to check your supplements against your medications.
4. **Work with your doctor.** Share your results and adjust dosages or timing for maximum benefit.
5. **Test regularly.** Start by rechecking your levels every 3–6 months to see how your body responds. Once your levels are where they should be, test at least yearly to make sure they stay that way.

CHAPTER 14

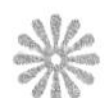

# PREVENTIVE MEDICINE AND LONGEVITY

Aging isn't a law of nature—it's a biochemical process we can influence. Just like we use antibiotics to treat infections and drugs to treat cancer, we can use science to slow down aging. Now, I didn't say it was easy, but we are getting better at slowing aging. Our cells change over time, affected most by sleep, diet, exercise, and stress, followed by hormone levels, genes, and environmental factors.

New tools like AI can help with this. Scientists can now track these changes in your body, from DNA damage to cells losing energy. They're also finding ways to slow aging down. This chapter shows how science and AI can help you stay healthy longer.

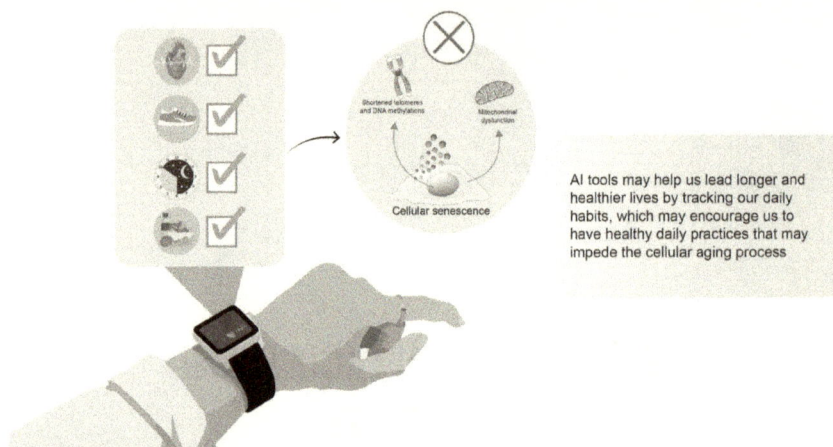

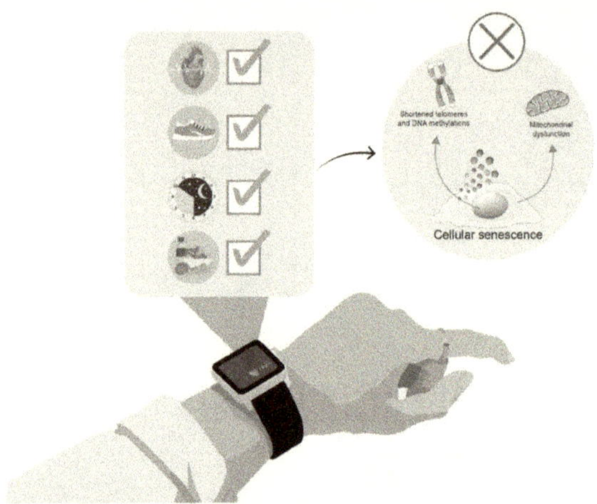


AI tools may help us lead longer and healthier lives by tracking our daily habits, which may encourage us to have healthy daily practices that may impede the cellular aging process

We'll also cover practical tips in the Body Hacks section at the end. Here's how it works:

Aging happens in three main ways: the protective tips on our DNA get shorter, our genes change in ways that speed up aging, and our cells lose energy (Sinclair & LaPlante, 2019). Think of it like a car—the protective coating wears off, the engine settings get mixed up, and the battery runs down.

To be more scientific... as we age, several things happen in our bodies at once. The protective caps on our chromosomes (telomeres) get shorter, like shoelaces losing their plastic tips. Our genes get chemical changes (epigenetic alterations) that affect how they work, like switches getting stuck in the wrong position. And our cells struggle to make energy efficiently, like a weakening battery.

Each of these changes affects the others, creating a cycle we're learning to slow down. Today, AI tools are getting better at tracking all three of these aging signs, helping doctors spot problems earlier than ever before.

Can we slow aging down, stop it, or turn it back? Science says we can influence it—more than I would have guessed

10 years ago. Aging is not some fixed law like gravity. It's a complex mix of biological shifts we're starting to measure and tweak. Medicines already change our body chemistry—insulin controls blood sugar and blood pressure medications protect your heart. Aging is more complex, but we're not helpless.

Our bodies don't just wear out like old machines. They change in specific ways we can now measure. As we age, damaged cells stick around and cause inflammation. Meanwhile, our stem cells—the body's repair team—slow down. Low-level inflammation slowly damages our tissues over time. That's aging—not a simple breakdown but changes we're learning to control.

We can measure these aging signs, but we don't fully understand how they work together. Lab studies don't always work in real people, and medical trials take years. Also, aging affects everyone differently. Your genes, lifestyle, and habits all matter. AI isn't smart enough yet to figure out all these personal factors at once.

Scientists are testing several ways to slow aging. Some approaches try to mimic the benefits of calorie restriction—eating significantly less than normal—which has extended lifespan in lab animals. The drug metformin, commonly used for diabetes, might provide these same benefits without the difficult diet. Another approach focuses on helping cells make energy more efficiently. Nutrients like CoQ10 and NAD+ boosters (a type of vitamin B) both support energy production in our cells.

New treatments called senolytics—a class of drugs that target specific cellular processes—work like a cleanup crew, removing old, damaged cells that cause inflammation and other problems. Another approach being tested is stem cell treatments, which use the body's own repair cells to fix damaged tissues. The National Institute on Aging tests these treatments through their research programs, including the Interventions Testing Program. So far, they show promise but no miraculous results yet.

### How AI Is Already Transforming Longevity Research

We've seen how AI wearables collect far more information than the occasional lab test or X-ray at the doctor's office. When it comes to longevity and extending our healthspan, this constant monitoring becomes especially powerful. The daily data about our sleep, exercise, and eating habits can help us make changes that lead to healthier, possibly longer lives.

I've seen patients transform after 6 months of healthier habits. AI can make these changes easier by using data from devices on our wrists to guide us. Studies show that personalized AI coaching helps people stick to healthy habits much better than general advice. This matters because consistency, not perfection, is what counts.

But here's an important caveat: AI is a tool, not the complete answer. A recent study on weight loss apps found something important—programs that combined human coaches with AI worked better than AI alone (Kapoor et al., 2025). Why? Human coaches bring something AI can't replicate: the power of real relationships. People try harder when they don't want to disappoint someone who's rooting for them. They show up because of friendship and accountability, not just data and reminders. AI can track everything perfectly and give smart suggestions, but it can't replace the feeling of having another person in your corner. The best results come when we use AI as a support tool while keeping the human connection that motivates us to actually make changes.

Sue, 51, felt exhausted despite normal bloodwork. She tested her aging markers and found low NAD+ and high inflammation. She started NMN supplements and improved her sleep. Six months later, her energy had soared, and tests showed better cellular health.

AI starts simple: tweaking sleep timing or flagging inflammation from diet. But the big win? All that data—heart rates, sleep cycles, food pics—builds a goldmine of information. AI could spot patterns we miss, like early metabolic shifts or lifestyle links to telomere health. In the future, AI might predict heart risks from meal timing or boost energy by optimizing daily walks.

While it's still early, the path is clear—aging is not the black box it once was, and AI is lighting it up. AI also supports simple health hacks, like morning light, to boost your healthspan (Wilson, 2025).

## Taking Action: What You Can Do Today

Try a wearable like Fitbit to track sleep, exercise, and diet, as described in Chapters 7 and 8. Consider trying AI-powered apps that can help with specific aspects of health:

- For sleep optimization, Sleep.ai and the Oura app offer insights based on your patterns
- Nutrition tracking apps like Lark and Foodvisor analyze your eating habits and suggest improvements
- For personalized workouts, apps like Fitbod and Future adapt to your progress and goals
- Meditation and stress apps such as Headspace and Calm can help manage the mental side of health

Choose apps with strong privacy policies, such as HIPAA-compliant or GDPR-certified platforms, to protect your health data. For instance, Oura's privacy policy ensures data encryption, but verify this for any app you use. Many of these tools offer free versions, though premium features may require payment.

When using these tools, focus on trends rather than daily fluctuations—look for patterns over weeks and months. Share relevant data with your healthcare provider by preparing summaries from your apps for more productive discussions.

Finally, stay informed but skeptical about longevity supplements and interventions. Follow reputable sources like the National Institute on Aging, Mayo Clinic, and Harvard Health Publishing for guidance based on solid science.

Diane, 44, was tired despite healthy habits. Her AI app flagged late meals and low protein, so she adjusted her diet. Two months later, her energy had surged, and her students noticed her vibrancy.

## The Future Is Just Beginning

Keep in mind that living longer is not the only goal. This is not just about more years. It's about more healthy years. Research on aging shows we can develop treatments that help people stay healthy as they age (Campisi et al., 2019). Scientists have studied something called compression of morbidity for over 40 years. This means squeezing the time of illness into a shorter period at the end of life. The goal is to add years of good health, not years of being sick (Fries et al., 2011).

We're moving from one-size-fits-all health advice to truly personalized medicine. AI is helping us understand that what works for your neighbor might not work for you, and that's okay. The future will likely bring even more sophisticated tools that can predict health issues before they happen and suggest interventions tailored to your unique biology. Stay curious, stay consistent, and watch your health transform.

### AI and Body Hacks for a Healthier, Happier You

My philosophy on health and medicine is simple: it's all about enjoying your life, not just avoiding sickness or chasing extra years. Too often, people twist health into something that steals their joy. A little discipline makes sense, but health should enhance your life, not control it.

Consider Bryan Johnson, a wealthy tech entrepreneur near Las Vegas. He has lowered his biological age 10–15 years through extreme measures like scheduling sex in a strict 90-minute window. It seems to work for him, but that level of control can strain relationships and drain the fun out of life. I would rather live with a bit more freedom and a lot more happiness.

Then there are people who force themselves into ice baths even when they hate them. Extreme steps like ice baths aren't needed for a healthier life. That said, building exercise habits, eating better, and sticking to a sleep schedule all seem reasonable. It is about balance, not punishment.

With that in mind, here are some practical, enjoyable body hacks and how AI can help you make them part of your life. The following is largely based on an excellent Audible Original by Kimberly Wilson titled *Hack Your Body, Heal Your Mind* (2025).

### Morning Light: A Simple Boost

Veronica, 45, felt happier after morning walks with AI app reminders. Science backs this up. Studies show that bright light therapy can improve depression symptoms significantly, with benefits often seen within 2 weeks of daily use (Golden et al., 2005). This makes morning light one of the best health investments for minimal effort.

Getting natural light in the morning helps in many ways. It can lift your mood, improve your sleep, and balance important hormones. These include melatonin (which controls sleep) and cortisol (which affects stress and energy). Neuroscientist Andrew Huberman (2022) explains that viewing bright light early in the day sets your body's internal clock for better sleep and mood.

The best time is within 1–3 hours of waking up. It's simple: step outside for 10 minutes with your coffee or take a short walk. No fancy tools needed. Just natural daylight on your face.

### How to Use This Hack with AI

Rise Science times your light exposure perfectly by analyzing your sleep data and local sunrise times. It suggests the best moment based on whether you're an early bird or night owl.

Google Assistant works with your calendar and local weather to send smart reminders: "It's sunny and you have 15 minutes before your meeting—perfect time for morning light."

The Sleep.ai app tracks improvements in your sleep quality and mood after consistent morning light exposure. Start by turning on location services on your phone. Set up a morning routine in your smart assistant using: "Remind me to get morning light when the weather is clear."

Track your sleep quality with Sleep Cycle or Oura Ring to see improvements.

## Sleep: Beyond Basic Rest

Sleep improves your health and can even lower your risk of getting dementia, as explained in Chapter 6. AI tools can help you get better sleep by tracking your patterns and suggesting changes.

### How to Use This Hack with AI

Sleep tracking devices can show you what's really happening when you sleep. The Oura Ring and Withings Sleep Analyzer track your deep sleep and REM sleep. These are the stages your brain and body need for recovery. The Eight Sleep Pod goes further: it changes your bed temperature through the night. It cools you down during deep sleep and warms you up before wake time.

Apps like SleepSpace can find patterns in your sleep data. They might discover that using your phone after 9 PM cuts your deep sleep by 20%. Or they might find that reading before bed increases it by 15%. These personal insights help you make better choices.

Start simple with a free app like Sleep Cycle. Use it for at least 2 weeks to gather data. Look at the app's analysis of your sleep patterns. Try its suggestions for bedtime, wake time, and bedroom setup. Track both your sleep scores and how you feel during the day.

New AI systems are being developed that can continuously learn from sleep data to provide smarter recommendations over time (Gamel & Talaat, 2024).

## Napping: Timing Is Everything

Naps can boost your energy, but timing matters. A 20-minute nap keeps you in light sleep—perfect for a quick pick-me-up. A 90-minute nap takes you through a full cycle, including deep and REM sleep, leaving you energized (Walker, 2017). Avoid 60 minutes though—waking from deep sleep feels awful.

### Quick Tips for Smart Napping

- Best timing: NapBot suggests when to nap based on your body's natural energy dips.

- Right length: Pzizz tracks your naps to learn if 20-minute power naps or 90-minute full cycles work better for you.
- Sleep tracking: Smart rings can tell when you actually fall asleep, not just when you lie down.
- Sound help: Brain.fm plays special sounds that help your brain relax for napping.

Try a nap app like Pzizz or NapBot to guide your rest. Start with 20 minutes and adjust based on how you feel. NASA research found that smart napping can boost your thinking by 34% and make you 54% more alert (Rosekind et al., 1995).

### Walking: Small Steps, Big Benefits

Alejandro, 50, eased stress with AI-guided walks after tough workdays. Walking sounds simple, but it's powerful. Just 10 minutes can calm stress, lift your mood, and get your body moving. Research shows that three 10-minute walks spread throughout the day work just as well as one 30-minute walk for improving fitness and lowering blood pressure (Murphy et al., 2009). Breaking up exercise into shorter chunks makes it easier to fit into busy schedules, which helps more people stick with their walking routine.

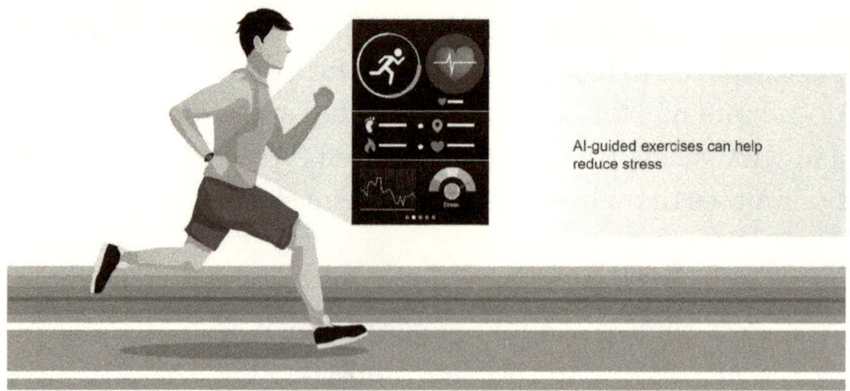

AI-guided exercises can help reduce stress

Since walking is weight-bearing, it's better for your bones and muscles than you might think. Out in nature, it's a mental reset. After a tough moment—like an argument with someone—a walk can cool you off.

### How to Use This Hack with AI

The Mindstrong app detects stress from typing patterns and voice tone before suggesting a brief walk. AllTrails and Strava recommend walking routes based on your preferences for terrain, greenery, or quiet areas. Fitbit Premium's AI discovers how different walking patterns (pace, duration, time of day) affect your particular stress markers and sleep quality. The Motion app identifies which meetings could be done while walking. Turn on notifications for your health app (Apple Health or Google Fit). Set up stress monitoring on your wearable device. Create a walking playlist that your AI assistant can trigger when needed.

## Metabolic Health: Catching Problems Early

Metabolic health, covered in Chapter 5, affects your weight and disease risk. AI now makes medical-grade tracking available to everyone. A study from Israel showed that personalized nutrition guided by AI cut blood sugar spikes after meals by 53% compared to standard diet advice (Zeevi et al., 2015).

### How to Use This Hack with AI

- Track food effects: The app Levels pairs with continuous glucose monitors to spot foods that raise blood sugar and suggest better choices.
- Analyze meals: Foodvisor checks meal photos and suggests small changes to improve how your body uses energy.

- Check energy use: Lumen measures your breath to see if you're burning carbs or fat.
- Spot issues early: MetricHealth uses wearable data to predict metabolic problems before standard tests. Start with a photo-based food app like Foodvisor. After 2 weeks, consider a CGM trial through Levels. Connect your activity data and review weekly insights about your metabolic responses.

## Hydration: The Overlooked Essential

Proper hydration affects everything from thinking clearly to muscle recovery. Yet most people rely on thirst, which only kicks in after you're already dehydrated. Research shows that being dehydrated by just 2% of your body weight hurts your ability to pay attention, remember things, and complete tasks (Adan, 2012). A review of 33 studies found that even mild dehydration slows down reaction times and makes it harder to focus, especially for tasks that need concentration (Wittbrodt & Millard-Stafford, 2018). Since your brain is about 75% water, it makes sense that losing even a small amount affects how well you think.

### Smart Hydration Steps

- Calculate needs: WaterMinder figures out your specific hydration needs based on weight, activity, and local temperature.
- Perfect timing: Hydration AI by Gatorade finds the best times to remind you when you're most likely to drink.
- See benefits: WHOOP strap connects hydration levels with recovery scores and workout performance.

- Early warning: When paired with Withings blood pressure monitors and fitness trackers, the Health Mate app can detect heart rate and blood pressure changes that may signal dehydration before you feel thirsty.

Try a hydration app like WaterMinder to monitor your water intake. Connect it to your health data for activity and environmental information. Log hydration for 2 weeks alongside mood and energy ratings.

## Play: The Fun Path to Health

Wei, 42, started painting after an AI app suggested it as a hobby, and she felt much happier. Kimberly Wilson (2025) makes a strong case for adult play—laughter, hobbies, travel—as vital to health. Play cuts stress, sparks creativity, and keeps your brain sharp. This fits my philosophy perfectly: health should feel good. Whether it's joking with friends, painting, exploring new places, playing with your dog, spending silly time with a child or grandchild, or being goofy with a fun-loving spouse, play is medicine you'll actually enjoy.

Research shows that playful adults handle stress better and report greater life satisfaction than less playful adults (Magnuson & Barnett, 2013). They also tend to be more active and do more enjoyable activities throughout their day (Proyer, 2013). Your brain literally changes when you play: new neural pathways form, creativity increases, and stress melts away.

### How to Use This Hack with AI

The Playtime AI app finds open blocks in your calendar and suggests playful activities matched to your personality. Daylio uses AI to connect your mood entries with activities, identifying which forms of play most reliably boost your mental state. Meetup learns your interests and suggests local playful social activities. The Oblique Strategies app generates creative prompts tailored to your interests when you're feeling stuck. Track your mood and activities with an app like Daylio for 2 weeks. Review the AI-generated connections between activities and positive moods. Schedule at least three play blocks in your calendar each week.

## Slow Breathing: Calm on Command

Slow, controlled breathing can lower stress, steady your heart, and clear your head. Research shows that 8 weeks of breathing exercises can reduce negative emotions and lower cortisol, your body's main stress hormone (Ma et al., 2017). Try breathing in for 4 seconds and out for 6 seconds. This type of breathing turns on your body's relaxation response, making it perfect for stressful moments. Anyone can do it, anywhere—no special equipment needed.

### How to Use This Hack with AI

- Detect stress: Spire Stone spots breathing patterns linked to stress and alerts you early.
- Find your rhythm: Breathwrk checks your heart rate changes to pick the best breathing pattern.
- Get real-time help: Breathe uses your phone's mic to guide your breathing as you go.
- Track progress: Wellory's AI shows how fast breathing calms your body's stress signals.

Download a breathing app like Breathwrk or Calm. Try the main protocols (4-7-8, box breathing, resonant breathing). Note which pattern works best for you in different situations.

## Hormesis: Stress That Strengthens You

Hormesis means small stresses can make your body stronger. Small doses of stress—like cold or heat—can toughen you up and boost immunity and resilience. But it's not for everyone, and AI can tailor it safely.

### Cold Exposure: Ice Baths and Showers

Cold showers or plunges kickstart hormesis—think better blood flow and stronger immune system. Hate them? Skip them—that's my philosophy! The Cold Plunge Coach app checks if cold exposure is safe for you. The Wim Hof Method app creates a gradual plan. Start with 15–30 seconds of cold at the end of your shower. Track your energy to monitor responses. Regular cold exposure can reduce inflammation markers and improve insulin sensitivity, with studies showing beneficial effects on immune function and metabolic health (Espeland et al., 2022).

### Heat Exposure: Saunas and More

Saunas or hot baths trigger heat shock proteins that help with cell repair and heart health. Consistency matters more than intensity. SaunaSpace can tailor sauna sessions to your goals. Smart watches can monitor your heart rate for safety. Start with 5–10 minutes at 150°F. Track how you feel afterward. Studies show that using a sauna four to seven times per week is linked to much lower risk of heart disease death compared to once-weekly use. The more often people used saunas, the better their heart health outcomes (Laukkanen et al., 2018).

### Fasting: Smart Nutrition Timing

Intermittent fasting has gained popularity for its metabolic benefits, but the optimal approach varies widely between individuals.

Before jumping into that trendy 16:8 fasting schedule AI recommended, let me share why Sally, a 45-year-old patient, was grateful she checked with me first. Her blood sugar tends to drop unexpectedly—something we discovered years ago when she nearly fainted at work. For her, skipping breakfast could mean passing out behind the wheel during her morning commute. We modified the plan: she does a gentler 12-hour fast and always keeps glucose tablets handy. Another patient with acid reflux found that fasting made his symptoms unbearable. We adjusted his eating window to work with his medication schedule. Your doctor knows your body's quirks from years of visits—information no AI has access to.

#### How to Use This Hack with AI

- Choose a fasting style: Zero's AI suggests a protocol (e.g., 16:8, 5:2) based on your health and goals.
- Find your eating window: Fast Habit picks the best time for you to eat based on your activity and energy.
- Stay on track: LIFE Fasting Tracker predicts when you might slip and offers support.

Start with simple time-restricted eating (12-hour window). Use a fasting app to track your eating periods. Note your energy levels and mood during and after fasts. Studies show that people who actively use fasting apps and track consistently achieve better weight loss results (Steger et al., 2022).

### Individual Differences Matter

While human biology is similar across populations, individual responses to these steps can vary significantly. AI's ability to analyze your personal data patterns makes it valuable for identifying which approaches work best for your unique body. FitnessGenes and DNAfit use AI to analyze genetic markers that might affect your response to fasting or cold exposure. Advanced health apps learn your cultural food preferences and suggest modifications that maintain traditional elements while improving health benefits. AI can modify recommendations based on your living situation—for example, suggesting indoor light therapy if outdoor walks aren't safe.

## Putting It All Together

The real power of AI comes when these health hacks work together in one system that changes with you. Ask AI to pick one or two hacks that will help you most based on your current health data, so you don't get overwhelmed with too many changes at once. When your life changes—like when you travel, get sick, or feel stressed—AI adjusts what it suggests to match what you can actually handle right now.

Start with a main health app like Apple Health, Google Fit, or Cronometer. Connect your fitness tracker or smartwatch. Pick just one hack that sounds good to you—getting morning sunlight is a great place to start. Once that becomes a habit, add a second step. Use what AI tells you to improve your approach based on how your own body responds.

## Wrapping Up

Health means feeling good, not perfection, as discussed in the chapter. These hacks, from morning light to playful moments, support that philosophy. AI makes them easier by analyzing your data to identify which approaches work best for your unique biology then helps you stick with them through timely reminders and progress tracking. The key advantage of AI in health improvement is not merely convenience but tailoring. Instead of following generic health advice, you can discover which specific steps produce the best results for your body. This makes the path to better health more efficient and enjoyable. Pick the hacks that resonate with you. Let AI help you use them intelligently. Remember that the goal is not to live forever. It is to live better right now.

CHAPTER 15

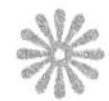

# AI AS YOUR HELPER

## AI as Your Research Partner

It is profoundly important to quickly access and analyze current evidence when making health decisions. AI tools excel at this task, helping you navigate complex medical literature and understand how research findings apply to your specific situation. Unlike human researchers who might take months to compile and analyze studies, AI can review hundreds of publications quickly and identify relevant patterns.

The goal isn't to replace medical expertise but to enhance the information available for medical decision-making. When you bring current research to healthcare discussions, you're not challenging your doctor's authority. Instead, you're making sure that decisions are based on the most complete evidence available. Most physicians welcome patients who come prepared with relevant research, as it shows engagement and can lead to more productive conversations about treatment options.

## Put AI to Work for Your Health: The Flipped Script Technique

Most people approach AI with direct questions: "What should I do about X?" But there's a more powerful technique that gets dramatically better results: the flipped script. Instead of asking AI for answers, you ask AI what questions you should be asking.

This simple shift transforms generic responses into personalized, comprehensive guidance. When you flip the script, AI becomes your strategic partner, helping you identify blind spots and considerations you never would have thought of on your own.

**The Standard Approach:** "I have [condition]. What should I do?"

**The Flipped Script:** "I have [condition]. What information do you need from me to give me the best guidance? What questions should I be asking you?"

This technique works because AI can draw from thousands of medical cases and research studies to find what matters most for your situation. It reveals questions about second opinions—not just on treatment plans but on original pathology slides. This matters because if the initial diagnosis is wrong, it changes everything. It considers practical factors like your location and which specialty centers are easiest to reach. It uncovers options you didn't know existed.

The following example shows this technique in action. The response is detailed—you can skim through it—but notice how much more complete and useful the flipped script response becomes compared to the basic approach. This level of detail can be the difference between getting standard care and getting the best possible care.

### Breast Cancer as an Example

Remember Anthony from the introduction, whose wife received a breast cancer diagnosis? Let me show you exactly how he used strategic questioning to get the detailed, personalized guidance that proved so valuable during that overwhelming time. This is long but note how much more detailed the flipped script response is. You can skim through it, but to Anthony and his wife, it was very important.

**Basic Prompt:** "My wife was just diagnosed with breast cancer. How can I get her the best care?"

### AI's Basic Response

"I'm sorry to hear about your wife's diagnosis. Here are some steps to ensure she gets quality care:

1. **Find a good oncologist.** Look for board-certified medical oncologists who specialize in breast cancer. You can search through your insurance network or ask for referrals from her primary care doctor.
2. **Consider comprehensive cancer centers.** Major hospitals often have dedicated breast cancer programs with multidisciplinary teams.
3. **Get a second opinion.** This is standard practice and most doctors encourage it, especially for cancer diagnoses.
4. **Research treatment options.** Learn about surgery, chemotherapy, radiation, and hormone therapy options that might apply to her case.
5. **Join support groups.** Organizations like the American Cancer Society offer resources for patients and families.

6. **Understand your insurance.** Make sure you know what's covered and any preauthorization requirements.
7. **Ask questions.** Don't hesitate to ask doctors to explain anything you don't understand.
8. **Keep organized records.** Maintain copies of all test results, treatment plans, and medical records.

The most important thing is to act quickly but not rush into decisions. Take time to understand her specific diagnosis and treatment options."

**The Flipped Script Prompt:** "My wife was just diagnosed with breast cancer. I want to get her the best care. What information do you need from me? What should I be asking you to help navigate this effectively?"

### AI's Response to the Flipped Script

"I can help you navigate this more effectively if you share some key details. Here's what would help me give you better guidance:

#### About the diagnosis

- What type and stage of breast cancer?
- What tests have been done so far (biopsy results, imaging)?
- Has she met with an oncologist yet?

#### About your situation

- Where are you located? (for finding specialists nearby)
- What's your insurance situation?
- Any family history of breast or ovarian cancer?
- Her age and general health status?

### What to ask me

- What questions should we ask the oncologist at our first appointment?
- What are the typical treatment timelines for [her specific type]?
- How do we evaluate if a treatment center is high-quality?
- What support resources exist for patients and families?
- What should we expect during treatment?

Would you like to start with any of these areas?"

### Anthony's Follow-Up Prompt Using AI's Suggestions

"She's 52, diagnosed with stage 2A invasive ductal carcinoma, ER/PR positive, HER2 negative. We're in Atlanta. She has good insurance through her employer. No family history. We meet the oncologist next Tuesday. What specific questions should we ask, and how do we know if we're getting the right treatment plan?"

### AI's Targeted Response

"Great—this gives me much better context. For stage 2A, ER/PR+ breast cancer, here are the key questions for Tuesday:

> Facing a diagnosis of stage 2A invasive ductal carcinoma (IDC), ER/PR-positive, HER2-negative is understandably overwhelming, but preparing for your oncologist meeting with targeted questions, ensuring an accurate pathology review, and considering a second opinion can help ensure your wife receives the best care. Below is a list of specific questions to ask your oncologist, guidance on evaluating

the treatment plan, advice on getting a second opinion on pathology slides, and considerations for seeking a second opinion at MD Anderson, tailored to your situation in Atlanta with good insurance and no family history.

### Questions to Ask the Oncologist

These questions will help clarify your wife's diagnosis, treatment options, and long-term care, focusing on her specific case (stage 2A IDC, ER/PR+, HER2−, no family history). They draw from expert recommendations and aim to empower you to understand the treatment rationale and align it with your wife's preferences.

About the Diagnosis

- Can you confirm the details of the pathology report?
  - Ask for specifics on tumor size, lymph node involvement (stage 2A typically means a tumor 2–5 cm with no lymph node spread or ≤2 cm with one to three positive lymph nodes), grade (how aggressive the cells look), and Ki-67 score (a measure of tumor growth rate). Confirm ER/PR positivity levels (e.g., percentage of receptors) and HER2 status, as these impact hormone therapy and treatment decisions.
  - Why this matters: This ensures you understand the tumor's characteristics, which drive treatment decisions.
- Should we get a second opinion on the pathology slides?
  - Request a second review of the pathology slides by another expert pathologist, ideally at a major cancer center like MD Anderson or Emory Winship Cancer

Institute in Atlanta. Pathology errors (e.g., misgrading or misinterpreting ER/PR/HER2 status) occur in ~10–20% of breast cancer cases and can significantly alter treatment plans.

- Why this matters: This confirms the diagnosis's accuracy, especially for ER/PR positivity and HER2 negativity, which dictate hormone therapy and chemotherapy decisions.

- Are additional tests needed to refine the diagnosis or treatment plan?
  - There's a test (Oncotype DX) that looks at your tumor's genes to predict if cancer might come back. If your cancer is fueled by hormones (which many are), this test helps decide if you really need chemotherapy or if hormone-blocking pills alone will work. Ask if imaging (e.g., MRI, PET scan) or genetic testing (e.g., *BRCA1/BRCA2*) is recommended, given no family history but potential for inherited mutations.
  - Why this matters: Genomic tests can personalize treatment, potentially sparing chemotherapy if the recurrence risk is low.
- What is the likelihood of recurrence based on these tumor characteristics?
  - Ask for an estimate of recurrence risk and how factors like ER/PR positivity and HER2 negativity influence prognosis. Stage 2A has a good prognosis (5-year survival ~87% if lymph nodes are involved, higher if not), but individual factors matter.
  - Why this matters: This helps you understand the long-term outlook and tailor follow-up care.

### About Treatment Options

- What are the recommended treatment options, and why?
  - Expect surgery (lumpectomy or mastectomy) as the primary treatment for stage 2A IDC, often followed by radiation if lumpectomy is chosen. Your type of breast cancer grows when exposed to estrogen. We can block this with daily pills for 5–10 years. The specific medication depends on whether you've gone through menopause—younger women usually take tamoxifen, while women past menopause take different drugs that work better for them. Ask if chemotherapy is recommended—stage 2A tumors >0.5 cm may benefit, especially if high-risk features (e.g., high grade or Ki-67) are present, but Oncotype DX results could rule it out.
  - Why this matters: This clarifies the rationale for each treatment and whether chemotherapy is necessary.
- What are the benefits and risks of lumpectomy versus mastectomy?
  - Ask how tumor size, location, and breast size affect surgical options. Discuss recurrence rates (similar for both procedures when followed by radiation for lumpectomy) and impact on survival. Inquire about sentinel lymph node biopsy and risks of lymphedema if lymph nodes are removed.
  - Why this matters: This helps weigh cosmetic, emotional, and medical factors in choosing surgery.
- Will radiation therapy be necessary, and what are the side effects?
  - Radiation is typically recommended after lumpectomy or if lymph nodes are involved post-mastectomy.

Ask about the duration (4–8 weeks), side effects (e.g., fatigue, skin changes), and impact on breast reconstruction if chosen.
    - Why this matters: This prepares you for the treatment timeline and potential side effects.
- What hormone therapy is recommended, and for how long?
    - Since the tumor is ER/PR+, hormone therapy is critical to reduce recurrence risk. Ask about specific drugs (e.g., tamoxifen, anastrozole), duration (5–10 years), and side effects (e.g., hot flashes, bone health). Inquire if newer drugs like CDK4/6 inhibitors (e.g., abemaciclib) are appropriate for high-risk cases.
    - Why this matters: Hormone therapy is a long-term commitment, and understanding its role is key.
- Are there clinical trials we should consider?
    - Ask about trials for stage 2A ER/PR+, HER2− breast cancer, especially those testing new hormone therapies or de-escalation strategies (e.g., omitting chemotherapy). MD Anderson and other centers often lead such trials.
    - Why this matters: Trials may offer access to cutting-edge treatments.

About Side Effects and Lifestyle

- How will treatments affect quality of life, and what support is available?
    - Discuss potential side effects (e.g., fatigue, menopausal symptoms, fertility concerns) and resources like fertility preservation, wigs for hair loss, or

lymphedema management. Ask about support groups or counseling in Atlanta.
    - Why this matters: This addresses emotional and physical impacts, especially for younger patients concerned about fertility.

- What lifestyle changes can reduce recurrence risk?
    - Inquire about diet, exercise, alcohol reduction, and smoking cessation to lower risk. Ask about follow-up care, including mammograms and monitoring schedules.
    - Why this matters: This empowers your wife to take proactive steps for her health.

About the Care Team and Logistics

- Who will be part of the treatment team, and how will care be coordinated?
    - Confirm the roles of the surgeon, medical oncologist, radiation oncologist, and other specialists (e.g., plastic surgeon for reconstruction). Ask how communication works between team members and with you.
    - Why this matters: This ensures seamless care and clarity on who to contact.
- How does my wife's overall health and menopausal status affect treatment?
    - Share her general health, medications, and menopausal status (pre- or postmenopausal), as these influence hormone therapy choices and chemotherapy tolerance.
    - Why this matters: This personalizes the treatment plan to her health profile.

### Advice on Getting a Second Opinion on Pathology Slides

A second opinion on the pathology slides is highly recommended to ensure the accuracy of your wife's diagnosis, as errors in pathology reports can significantly impact treatment decisions. Here's how to approach it:

- Why it's important: Think of your pathology slides like an X-ray that needs to be read—except instead of looking at bones, pathologists are examining tiny pieces of tissue under a microscope to determine if cancer is present and what type it might be. Here's something most people don't realize: even experienced pathologists can disagree about what they're seeing. A recent review found that in some types of tissue samples—particularly from gynecology, skin, and digestive system biopsies—diagnostic errors occurred in more than 20% of cases (Peck et al., 2018). That doesn't mean your pathologist is incompetent; it means that interpreting these tissue samples can be genuinely challenging, like trying to identify a specific type of tree from just a few leaves. The good news is that getting a second expert to review your slides dramatically reduces the chance of error. Just as you wouldn't hesitate to get a second opinion on a treatment plan, having another pathologist review the actual tissue samples ensures that the foundation of your diagnosis—and therefore your entire treatment plan—is as accurate as possible.

  Pathology slides determine critical details like tumor type (IDC), stage (2A), grade, and receptor status (ER/PR+, HER2−). Studies show discrepancies in ~10–20% of breast cancer pathology reports, particularly in hormone receptor or HER2 status, which could lead to incorrect treatments (e.g., omitting hormone therapy if ER/PR status is misread). A second review by an expert pathologist reduces this risk.

- How to arrange it: Ask your current hospital or oncologist to send the pathology slides to a major cancer center, such as MD Anderson's Breast Pathology Department or Emory Winship Cancer Institute in Atlanta. MD Anderson offers pathology second opinions, often remotely, requiring only the slides and pathology report. Contact MD Anderson (1-877-632-6789 or www.mdanderson.org) or Emory (404-778-7777) to initiate the process. Your wife's insurance should cover this but confirm with the provider.
- Who should review: Choose a center with specialized breast pathologists, as they have expertise in interpreting subtle differences in IDC and receptor status. MD Anderson is renowned for its pathology department, but Emory is a strong local option.
- Timing: Request the second opinion promptly, ideally before your Tuesday meeting or shortly after, to avoid delaying treatment. Pathology reviews typically take a few days to a week.
- What to ask: When discussing results, ask the reviewing pathologist to confirm tumor size, grade, lymph node status, ER/PR percentage, HER2 status, and any discrepancies with the original report. Ensure the oncologist integrates these findings into the treatment plan.

### Evaluating the Treatment Plan

To determine if the treatment plan is appropriate, consider these factors:

- Alignment with guidelines: The plan should align with National Comprehensive Cancer Network (NCCN) guidelines, which recommend surgery (lumpectomy or mastectomy) for stage 2A IDC, followed by radiation for lumpectomy or, if lymph nodes are involved, hormone therapy for ER/PR+ tumors, and chemotherapy based on tumor size, grade, or Oncotype DX score.
- Pathology accuracy: Ensure the plan is based on a verified pathology report. If a second pathology opinion reveals discrepancies (e.g., incorrect ER/PR status), the treatment plan may need adjustment.
- Personalization: The plan should reflect tumor characteristics (e.g., low Oncotype DX score may avoid chemo) and your wife's preferences (e.g., breast conservation versus mastectomy).
- Transparency: The oncologist should explain why each treatment is recommended, supported by pathology and test results. If chemotherapy is suggested, ask for the Oncotype DX score or other evidence justifying it.
- Comprehensive care: The plan should include side effect management, follow-up schedules (e.g., mammograms every 6–12 months), and support services.
- Prognosis discussion: The oncologist should provide a clear prognosis (stage 2A ER/PR+, HER2− typically has a good outlook with proper treatment) and address recurrence risks.

If the plan feels rushed or unclear, doesn't address test result conflicts, or dismisses your concerns, these are red flags. A good plan balances evidence-based care with your wife's values (e.g., preserving fertility, minimizing side effects).

Seeking a second opinion at MD Anderson Cancer Center is a reasonable and potentially valuable step, especially given your proximity (direct flight from Atlanta), good insurance, and the importance of confirming the pathology and treatment plan. Here's why and how to approach it:

### Benefits of a Second Opinion

- Expertise: MD Anderson is a top-ranked cancer center with extensive experience in breast cancer, including stage 2A IDC. Their breast pathologists can provide a definitive second opinion on the pathology slides, and their oncologists can refine the treatment plan (e.g., confirming if chemo is needed via genomic testing).
- Confirmation or adjustment: A second opinion can confirm the initial plan or suggest alternatives (e.g., a less aggressive approach if Oncotype DX indicates low recurrence risk). About 1–10% of second opinions lead to significant treatment changes, such as adjusting surgery or systemic therapy.
- Pathology review: MD Anderson's pathology department can reevaluate the slides to ensure accuracy in tumor characteristics and receptor status, which is critical for ER/PR+, HER2− tumors.
- Access to trials: MD Anderson offers trials for ER/PR+, HER2− cancers, which could provide innovative options.

- Peace of mind: Even if the plan remains unchanged, a second opinion, including pathology review, can increase confidence in the approach, especially for a life-altering diagnosis.

Logistics

- Insurance: Your wife's good employer-based insurance likely covers second opinions, including pathology reviews, but confirm with the provider whether MD Anderson (Houston, TX) is in-network or if out-of-network benefits apply. Contact MD Anderson's patient access team (1-877-632-6789 or www.mdanderson.org) to verify coverage and costs for both the clinical consultation and pathology review.
- Process: Request a second opinion through MD Anderson's Breast Cancer Center. Provide medical records, pathology slides, and imaging. The pathology review can often be done remotely, while the clinical consultation may be remote or in-person. A second opinion typically takes a few days to a week, which won't significantly delay treatment.
- Travel: Direct flights from Atlanta to Houston (e.g., Delta, United) take ~2 hours and cost $200–500 round-trip, depending on booking. MD Anderson offers patient travel support services, including lodging recommendations. Check with your insurance for travel reimbursement if applicable.
- Timing: Schedule the second opinion, including pathology review, soon, ideally before starting treatment, but after your Tuesday meeting to compare recommendations. If surgery is urgent (e.g., aggressive tumor),

request expedited pathology review, which MD Anderson can often complete within 24–48 hours."

**The Difference:** The basic prompt gave generic advice that applies to anyone with cancer. The flipped script transformed the conversation into actionable, personalized guidance that directly addresses their specific situation—exactly the kind of detailed guidance Anthony and his wife needed.

The key insight is that AI's real power isn't in giving you quick answers—it's in helping you ask better questions. Whether you're dealing with a new diagnosis, considering genetic testing, or planning prevention strategies, this approach transforms AI from a simple search tool into a strategic health advisor that provides the specific, actionable guidance you need most.

As you apply these techniques with data from wearables, lab results, genetic tests, and medical records, you'll discover insights that would otherwise remain hidden. Use AI systems with broad medical knowledge rather than narrow specialty apps unless you have a specific condition.

AI serves as your research assistant, helping you access current medical literature, understand complex data, and advocate effectively for your health. When healthcare systems move slowly, when financial pressures create barriers, or when agreement proves incomplete, these tools give you the power to participate meaningfully in your healthcare decisions. You deserve access to complete, current information when making choices that affect your health and quality of life.

One of the biggest headaches patients face—beyond their actual health problems—is making sense of confusing medical bills. Hospital bills are often filled with codes and charges that seem designed to confuse rather than clarify. Here's where AI can really help. You can scan your medical bill, upload it as a PDF, and ask AI to look for problems. Recently, a family did exactly this after receiving a $195,000 bill for their relative's final 4 hours of care after a heart attack. They uploaded the bill to Claude AI and asked it to analyze the charges. What the AI found was troubling: the hospital had billed them twice for the same procedures—once for the "master procedure" and then again for every single step within it. That double-billing alone added up to about $100,000. The AI also spotted improper coding and billing violations, like charging for ventilator services on the same day as an emergency admission, which isn't allowed under Medicare rules (Tyson, 2025). With AI's help writing clear, professional letters pointing out these errors, the family got the bill reduced to $33,000.

Here's what this story teaches us: hospitals sometimes count on patients not knowing enough to question their bills. But you don't need to be a billing expert anymore. AI can analyze your bills the same way it analyzes your lab results or research papers. Upload your itemized bill and ask the AI to look for duplicate charges, coding errors, or charges that are higher than what Medicare would pay. The AI can even help you write professional letters to dispute wrong charges. Think of it as having a knowledgeable friend who understands medical billing sitting with you at your kitchen table, going through everything line by line. Will every bill have errors? No. But when they do, you'll catch them. As the family in this case put it, "Nobody should pay more out of pocket than Medicare would pay" (Tyson, 2025, para. 16). AI helps make sure that happens.

The future of healthcare lies not in replacing human expertise with artificial intelligence but in combining the analytical power of AI with the wisdom, experience, and compassion of healthcare professionals. By learning to use these tools effectively, you become a more informed participant in your healthcare journey, better equipped to navigate the complexities of modern medicine and advocate for the care you need.

Always consult with healthcare professionals when using AI health tools. These tools support medical care but don't replace professional medical advice.

The future of personal health is in your hands. Use this approach, and you'll never look at your health data the same way again.

CONCLUSION

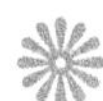

# THE COMING REVOLUTION IN PERSONAL HEALTH

## AI and Health—From Promise to Practice

The past 10 years have been amazing. We've gone from basic step counters to full health monitors. Paper vaccine records changed to digital tracking. Guessing about vitamins was replaced by science-based advice. Most importantly, we now prevent illness before it starts.

This shift is more than technology. It's a new way to think about health. Healthcare used to be something doctors did to fix you when you got sick, but now it's something you do every day to stay healthy. AI makes this work by turning complex body information into simple insights you can use.

## Technology That Serves Life

As I have said, my approach in treating patients has been simple: health technology should help us enjoy life. It should not burden us with too many rules. Basic habits like good sleep, moving your body, and eating well are not too much to ask. These basics give us energy to enjoy life fully.

Technology must serve life, not control it. Even the most advanced brain interface or tiny sensor is worthless if it doesn't make our lives better. We need to ask not just "What can this do?" but "How does this make life more enjoyable?"

As our devices collect more personal body data, we need better privacy protection. Everyone should understand what data are collected, how they're used, and who can access them.

## Your Next Steps

This book invites you to help shape how technology improves your health. Here are simple steps:

Start with what's already available. Use the health app on your phone or websites that look at your lab results. Many require no equipment and cost nothing.

Focus on basics first: sleep, exercise, nutrition, and stress management. Even advanced technology cannot make up for ignoring these foundations.

Approach health monitoring with curiosity, not worry. The goal is insight, not stress.

Consider sharing your anonymous health data for research. Programs like All of Us Research Program accept data. Your information could help develop tools that save lives.

Support efforts that extend these technologies to underserved communities. Health innovation should benefit everyone.

**Important:** Always talk to healthcare professionals when using AI health tools. These tools support medical care but don't replace professional advice.

## What's Coming Next

### Smart Health Monitoring

Predicting AI's health future is like forecasting weather—we can see patterns, but details stay unclear. I've seen technology save lives in real time. One patient's wearable device caught a dangerous heart rhythm before she felt symptoms. This allowed treatment before a heart attack. The future makes these abilities much stronger.

AI will monitor your body continuously through devices from wearables to implants. It will even analyze molecules you breathe out. This isn't about replacing doctors. It's about catching problems early when they're easiest to treat.

Today's wearables will keep getting better. They'll be joined by smart sensors that shrink from pea-sized to microscopic. Blood testing will evolve from checking a few markers (biological clues your body gives about your health) to telling your complete biological story.

### Better Wearables

By 2030, wearable devices will track much more than just your steps and heart rate. New sensors will measure stress hormones like cortisol right from your sweat, giving you instant feedback about how stressed your body is. Scientists at UCLA have already made a smartwatch that checks cortisol levels in sweat as well as a blood test can, but without any needles (Zhao et al., 2022). When cortisol touches special DNA sensors in the device, it creates an electrical signal that shows exactly how stressed you are.

This technology could help people with depression, anxiety, or PTSD track their condition all day long. Studies show these monitoring systems can help lower stress symptoms by alerting people when to do breathing exercises or relaxation techniques (An et al., 2022).

Earlier in this book, we explored how wearables can detect heart problems in people like Sarah, whose Apple Watch caught concerning patterns before she felt any symptoms. That technology keeps getting better. While basic smartwatches can track your pulse, newer devices do much more. They can spot AFib—an irregular heartbeat that causes many strokes—even when you don't feel it. With older watches, you'd need to remember to place your finger on the device for a 30-second ECG reading. But as we learned, AFib often has no symptoms. If you feel fine, why would you check? That's the problem with waiting for symptoms.

Apple Watch Series 4 and later models solve this by checking your pulse automatically throughout the day when you're sitting still. According to Apple, the watch looks for at least five rhythm checks over a minimum of 65 minutes, and if enough show irregular patterns, it alerts you about possible AFib—a feature that's been FDA-cleared since 2018 (Apple Inc., 2024). Studies confirm these smartwatches can detect AFib with 97–100% accuracy compared to medical ECG devices (Nazarian et al., 2021). This background monitoring catches AFib that would otherwise go unnoticed, potentially preventing strokes.

The technology isn't perfect yet—it only works when you're still and checks periodically rather than continuously. But it's already saving lives by finding problems people never knew they had. This background monitoring catches AFib that would otherwise go unnoticed, potentially preventing strokes.

The next advances will be even more powerful. Future wearables will monitor every heartbeat continuously, even during exercise. As we saw with Sarah's case, AI can already spot subtle heart problems through pattern analysis. New systems can find people whose hearts are pumping weakly before any symptoms appear—working like smoke detectors that smell trouble before you see flames (Attia et al., 2019). Soon, your watch will serve as a round-the-clock guardian, alerting you to developing problems weeks or months early. This gives you precious time to see a doctor and prevent heart attacks or strokes, just as Sarah's early warning led to life-saving treatment.

Sleep tracking is moving beyond just measuring sleep stages. Future wearables will detect breathing problems, teeth grinding, and early signs of sleep apnea without needing a full sleep study. They'll also track how your sleep affects your blood sugar, stress hormones, and immune system throughout the night. Some devices will even adjust your bedroom temperature and lighting automatically to improve sleep quality. With prices from $100–300, these devices are the easiest way for most people to try health AI.

### Invisible Implants

Implanted monitoring technology is becoming invisible. Today's implantable loop recorders—tiny devices doctors place just under the skin on your chest near your heart to track heart rhythms—are about the size of a USB flash drive or an average-sized paperclip but thicker. Within 5 years, they'll shrink to rice-grain size.

CGMs are already transforming diabetes care for 34 million Americans. Today's sensors stick to your skin for 2 weeks, tracking blood sugar without finger pricks. AI analyzes this data to predict problems and suggest food swaps that improve control by about 30%.

The next generation of CGMs will be even better. Future versions will be implanted completely under the skin—no more adhesive patches that can fall off during showers or exercise. These implanted devices will be smaller than today's dime-sized sensors, perhaps shrinking to rice-grain size within 5 years. Instead of replacing them every 2 weeks, they'll last 3 to 6 months before needing replacement. The needle insertion will become painless with new micro-needle technology. Data accuracy will improve, and AI predictions will become even more precise, potentially preventing 50% more blood sugar spikes than current systems.

Artificial pancreas systems—devices that automatically manage insulin for people with diabetes—are evolving from reactive to predictive devices. They learn your personal patterns and give you insulin automatically throughout the day. Studies show they can reduce dangerous blood sugar swings by 40–50% based on early research. Within the next decade, these systems will become smaller and smarter.

The next generation of health sensors will track much more than today's devices. They'll measure oxygen in your blood continuously, detect inflammation before you feel sick, and even spot proteins that appear when cancer cells first start growing. These advances are showing promise in early studies, though we're still measuring exactly how much earlier they'll catch diseases compared to current methods. These technologies could improve early detection by 20–40% compared to current methods, based on early studies.

### Blood Tests Tell Stories

Today's blood tests check limited markers—cholesterol, vitamins, basic panels. Tomorrow's blood analysis will tell your complete biological story through assessment of hormones, proteins, and genetic markers (biological codes that shape your health).

Gene testing—analyzing how your genes affect medication response—will become standard practice, potentially reducing bad drug reactions by 20–30% according to current research.

Most importantly, advanced blood tests will detect subtle inflammation markers and immune activity years before symptoms develop. These tests can identify different types of health problems much earlier than current methods.

For heart disease, a major study of nearly 28,000 women found that measuring inflammation markers like C-reactive protein (CRP) can predict risk up to 30 years in advance. Women with the highest CRP levels had a 70% increased risk of heart disease compared to those with the lowest levels (Ridker et al., 2024).

For mental health, researchers found that inflammation markers can predict depression and other mental disorders before symptoms appear, helping doctors identify people who might need early support (Huang et al., 2025). While the cost—roughly $200 annually—may seem high, avoiding expensive treatments makes this cost-effective.

## Emerging Technologies

In labs at Harvard, MIT, and other institutions, technologies that once seemed impossible are advancing rapidly. Sweat sensors already monitor glucose and stress hormones continuously.

Perhaps most futuristic is environmental DNA detection—sensors that analyze genetic material shed through your skin cells into the air around you. Think of it like leaving invisible fingerprints wherever you go. Early research suggests these could detect prediabetes from air samples 40–50% faster than blood tests.

Breath analysis offers another frontier. Devices can read biological clues in your exhaled air—like getting a health report from your breath—to spot lung problems and early cancer signs with 30% greater precision than current tools.

### Brain-Computer Connections

The most incredible breakthrough of all involves direct interfaces between brains and computers. Elon Musk's Neuralink has already implanted working prototypes in human patients. The coin-sized device, implanted through minor surgery, enabled a paralyzed person to play chess using only thoughts.

Neural interfaces could track brain activity patterns linked to dementia, epilepsy, or depression, potentially identifying these conditions 50–60% earlier than current diagnosis based on early research. Current neural interfaces require surgery, but noninvasive options may emerge by the 2030s.

## Promise Versus Reality

There's growing speculation that AI will cure all disease within 10 years. Some researchers predict a medical revolution like the discovery of antibiotics—a breakthrough that suddenly made deadly infections curable and added decades to human lifespans. Companies like DeepMind have shown AI can significantly speed drug discovery.

With my years of clinical practice, I am skeptical of such predictions. People will continue making self-destructive choices—overworking, neglecting self-care, self-medicating. Sometimes for understandable reasons, sometimes for ones that baffle physicians. Human behavior complexities won't disappear with technology.

However, 2025–2035 will likely bring the most dramatic changes in medicine since DNA's discovery. AI will transform how we prevent, detect, and treat disease.

## Ethical Concerns

The biggest challenge involves fair access. Advanced systems will likely reach wealthy communities first, potentially widening health gaps. However, healthcare systems waste about 20–30% of their spending on things like unnecessary procedures and inefficient care. AI could help eliminate much of this waste through prevention and early detection, making these technologies more accessible over time (World Economic Forum, 2018).

We must also address risks of biased AI algorithms that might work better for some groups than others. Patients can advocate for fair AI by asking companies how their tools are tested for diverse groups. These challenges require careful attention as technology advances.

## The Future We're Building

AI and healthcare are changing medicine and our relationship with our bodies. We're shifting from passive patients relying on experts to active participants understanding our own biology and preventing illness before it starts. This represents one of the most significant shifts in modern medicine.

The healthcare revolution driven by AI has just begun. Each year, these systems will become more accurate, less invasive, more accessible, and more personalized. AI health monitoring has real potential to transform healthcare in the 21st century—though likely not in the exaggerated timelines some predict. But this revolution offers something more valuable than extra years: it promises better years with less suffering.

Your journey to better health through AI doesn't require waiting. It starts with your next choice. Maybe downloading a health app, scheduling a blood test, or simply paying attention to what your body tells you every day.

The promise of AI in healthcare isn't about algorithms or sensors. It isn't about technology replacing human judgment or medical expertise. It's about empowering you with knowledge, catching problems early, and helping you make informed decisions about your health. It's about freeing human potential for what matters most. It's about creating conditions where we can thrive physically, emotionally, and spiritually. Not just for ourselves but for our loved ones, our friends, and our communities.

This is the future we're building together, and it begins now.

# Appendices

APPENDIX A

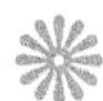

# MUST-HAVE LISTS TO TAKE TO EVERY MEDICAL APPOINTMENT

## REMEMBER TO BRING YOUR ID AND HEALTH INSURANCE CARD(S) TO EVERY APPOINTMENT

### Instructions

Print this form and complete it before each medical appointment. Keep it updated as your medications, supplements, or health status change. Consider bringing both a paper copy and a digital version, as internet access can be unreliable in medical facilities, and most healthcare providers will not download files from patients for security reasons.

### DIAGNOSES/MEDICAL CONDITIONS

| Diagnosis/ Condition | When Diagnosed | Treating Physician | Current Status |
|---|---|---|---|
| | | | |
| | | | |
| | | | |
| | | | |

*Add additional rows as needed*

## MEDICATION LIST

| Medication Name | Route (oral, inject, topical) | Strength (mg, mcg, %) | Times Per Day | When Taken (specific times) | Daily or As Needed? | If As Needed, When? |
|---|---|---|---|---|---|---|
| | | | | | | |
| | | | | | | |
| | | | | | | |
| | | | | | | |
| | | | | | | |
| | | | | | | |
| | | | | | | |

*Add additional rows as needed*

## MEDICATION ALLERGIES

| Drug Name | Reaction/ Symptoms | When Did This Happen? | Personally Experienced or Reported by Others? |
|---|---|---|---|
| | | | |
| | | | |
| | | | |

*Add additional rows as needed*

## SUPPLEMENT LIST

| Supplement Name | Form (tablet, capsule, liquid) | Strength | Times Per Day | When Taken | Brand | Reason for Taking |
|---|---|---|---|---|---|---|
| | | | | | | |
| | | | | | | |
| | | | | | | |

| Supplement Name | Form (tablet, capsule, liquid) | Strength | Times Per Day | When Taken | Brand | Reason for Taking |
|---|---|---|---|---|---|---|
| | | | | | | |
| | | | | | | |
| | | | | | | |

*Add additional rows as needed*

## Important Additional Information

### Recent Hospitalizations or Emergency Room Visits

| Date | Reason | Hospital/Facility | Treating Physician |
|---|---|---|---|
| | | | |
| | | | |

### Previous Surgeries

| Date | Surgery Type | Hospital/Facility | Surgeon |
|---|---|---|---|
| | | | |
| | | | |
| | | | |

Last Updated: ____________________________ (date)

## PHARMACOGENOMIC TEST RESULTS

If you have had pharmacogenomic testing, attach your lab results directly to this form. These tests show how your body metabolizes various medications based on your genetic profile. The following genes are particularly relevant to medication metabolism:

| Gene | Your Result | Clinical Significance |
|---|---|---|
| *CYP2D6* | | Affects metabolism of many antidepressants, antipsychotics, beta-blockers, and opioid pain medications |
| *CYP2C19* | | Affects metabolism of proton pump inhibitors, antidepressants, antiepileptics, and antiplatelet drugs |
| *CYP2C9* | | Affects metabolism of NSAIDs, sulfonylureas, and warfarin |
| *CYP3A4/5* | | Affects metabolism of statins, benzodiazepines, and many other drugs |
| *VKORC1* | | Affects response to warfarin |
| *SLCO1B1* | | Affects statin metabolism and risk of side effects |
| *HLA-B*15:02* | | Associated with severe skin reactions to certain antiepileptic drugs |
| *HLA-B*57:01* | | Associated with hypersensitivity to abacavir |
| *TPMT* | | Affects metabolism of thiopurines |
| *DPYD* | | Affects metabolism of fluoropyrimidines used in cancer treatment |
| *UGT1A1* | | Affects metabolism of irinotecan and other drugs |
| *G6PD* | | Can lead to hemolytic anemia with certain drugs |

*Note: Not all pharmacogenomic tests include all these genes. Only list the ones included in your test results.*

APPENDIX B

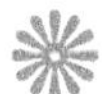

# GETTING DATA FROM YOUR WEARABLES (APPLE IOS USERS)

Wearable technology evolves quickly, with new models and improved methods of data access appearing regularly. While I provide current export instructions for popular devices below, these steps might change as companies update their apps and services. For the most up-to-date method specific to your device, try asking an AI assistant: "I have a [your specific device name and model]. What is the current method to export my [specific data like sleep, heart rate, etc.] data into a format I can analyze or share with my doctor? Please include step-by-step instructions using the latest apps and features." This ensures you'll always have current guidance, even as technology advances.

If you're an iPhone user, your wearable data are a goldmine for understanding sleep, fitness, and recovery. Here's how to pull that info from your device, save it as an Excel file, and feed it to an AI like Grok 3 for smart insights. Each wearable has its quirks, so I've tailored the steps below.

### Before You Start: Exporting from Apple Health

Most iOS wearables sync with Apple Health, so here's the universal trick to grab your data:

- Open the **Health app** on your iPhone.
- Tap **Sources** > Select your device > Choose **Export All Health Data**. (It'll save as an XML file.)
- Convert it to a CSV (Excel-friendly) file using a free app like "Health Export" or "QS Access" from the App Store. Open the CSV file in Excel and save as .xlsx.
- **Uploading**: For Grok 3, copy-paste up to 1–2 years of data into a query. For other AIs, use their "Attach File" option.

Now, let's dive into your options.

### 1. Apple Watch Series 10

- **Why It's Great:** The fitness champ—real-time heart rate, ECG, and workout tracking, plus decent sleep stats. Perfect if you're active and prefer Apple devices.
- **Quick Tip:** Charge it nightly and watch for sleep apnea alerts in 2025.

**How to Download Data**

- Open the **Health app** and follow the Before You Start steps, above. Your sleep stages, heart rate, and activity data are all there.
- Done! You've got an Excel file ready to go.

**Tell the AI**

- "Look at my Apple Watch data from [date range, up to 1–2 years]. Check sleep stages, workout heart rates, and activity trends. Spot any red flags (like low sleep or high heart rate) and give me two or three easy tweaks for better fitness and rest."

2. Oura Ring 4

- **Why It's Great:** The sleep-tracking king—deep, REM, light stages, plus HRV and readiness scores. Sleek titanium, 6–7-day battery—it's a lifestyle game-changer.
- **Quick Tip:** Wear it 24/7 to see how sleep impacts your energy. The $5.99/month subscription unlocks the full magic.

### How to Download Data

- Open the **Oura app** on your iPhone.
- Go to **Settings > Data Sharing > Apple Health** and turn on all categories (Sleep, Heart Rate, Activity).
- Follow the Before You Start steps, above, to export from Apple Health into Excel.

### Tell the AI

- "Dive into my Oura Ring 4 data from [date range, up to 1–2 years]. Focus on sleep stages, HRV, and readiness. Link low HRV or bad sleep to specific times, and suggest two or three steps to boost recovery."

3. RingConn Gen 2

- **Why It's Great:** Budget-friendly ($279), no subscription, and a whopping 12-day battery. Covers sleep, HRV, and steps—perfect for simplicity lovers.
- **Quick Tip:** Great starter if you're cost-conscious but want solid basics.

### How to Download Data

- Open the **RingConn app** on your iPhone.
- Hit **Settings > Apple Health** and enable data sharing.
- Use the Before You Start steps, above, to pull it from Apple Health into Excel.

### Tell the AI

- "Check my RingConn Gen 2 data from [date range, up to 1–2 years]. Focus on sleep quality and HRV trends. Give me two or three simple ideas to improve sleep or cut stress."

4. Whoop 4.0

- **Why It's Great:** A recovery beast—HRV, strain, and sleep stats for fitness buffs or chronic illness trackers. Five-day battery, comfy strap.
- **Quick Tip:** The $30/month subscription is worth it if you're serious about strain and rest.

### How to Download Data

- Open the **Whoop app** on your iPhone.
- Go to **Profile > More > Export Data**, pick your date range (up to 1–2 years), and get a CSV file emailed to you.
- Open the CSV file in Excel and save as .xlsx—no Apple Health detour needed!

### Tell the AI

- "Analyze my Whoop 4.0 data from [date range, up to 1–2 years]. Zero in on HRV, strain, and sleep. Pinpoint low-recovery stretches and recommend two or three ways to balance effort and rest."

## APPENDIX C

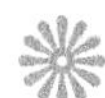

# INTEGRATING GENETIC DATA WITH OTHER HEALTH INFORMATION FOR AI ANALYSIS

Genetic testing technology and services evolve rapidly, with new options appearing regularly. While the instructions below reflect current methods for popular testing services, you can always get the most up-to-date guidance by asking an AI assistant: “What are the current options for accessing and downloading my raw genetic data from [name of testing company]? What are the best current tools for analyzing this genetic data for health insights?” This approach ensures you’ll have the latest information specific to the genetic testing service you used.

This appendix provides practical steps for combining your genetic test results with data from wearables, medication lists, and other health information so AI can provide more personalized insights.

### Getting Your Genetic Data Ready

Different genetic testing companies provide results in various formats. Here's how to access and prepare data from the most common services:

#### From Consumer Genetic Tests (23andMe, AncestryDNA)

1. **Download your raw data**
   - **23andMe:** Log in → Browse Raw Data → Download
   - **AncestryDNA:** Log in → Settings → DNA → Download Raw DNA Data
   - This will typically provide a .txt or .csv file
2. **Download your health reports**
   - Take screenshots or save PDFs of any health-related reports
   - For 23andMe: Health → Health Predispositions → Download PDF for each report

#### From Advanced Genetic Services (Nebula Genomics, New Amsterdam Genomics)

1. **Request a summary report.** Most comprehensive testing services provide summary reports designed to share with healthcare providers.
2. **Ask about AI-compatible exports.** Some services now offer exports formatted for AI analysis. Request this option if available.

## Creating a Unified Health Profile

### Method 1: Simple PDF Collection (Beginner-Friendly)

This method requires no technical skills and works with any AI that can process PDFs.

1. **Gather your documents**
   - Genetic test summary reports
   - Screenshots of important genetic variants
   - Recent lab work (blood tests, etc.)
   - Medication and supplement list
   - Wearable data summaries (export weekly or monthly reports)
2. **Create a single PDF**
   - Scan physical documents if needed
   - Combine all digital documents into one PDF using a free tool like Adobe Acrobat Reader (File → Create → Combine Files into Single PDF)
   - Alternatively, print everything and scan it as a single document
3. **Create a simple cover page** with the following:
   - Your age and sex
   - Major health concerns
   - Family history highlights
   - Main questions you want the AI to address

### Method 2: Structured Text File (Intermediate)

This method creates a more organized text file that AI can process more effectively.

1. **Create a text document** (.txt or .docx) with the following sections:

   PERSONAL INFORMATION

   Age: [Your age]

   Sex: [Your sex]

   Height: [Your height]

   Weight: [Your weight]

   Primary Health Concerns: [List your concerns]

   GENETIC HIGHLIGHTS

   Important Variants: [List key variants, e.g., *APOE* ε4/ε3, *MTHFR* C677T heterozygous]

   Pharmacogenomic Markers: [List drug metabolism genes, e.g., CYP2D6 *1/*4 - intermediate metabolizer]

   MEDICATION LIST

   [Medication Name] - [Dosage] - [Frequency]

   [Medication Name] - [Dosage] - [Frequency]

   SUPPLEMENT LIST

   [Supplement Name] - [Dosage] - [Frequency]

   [Supplement Name] - [Dosage] - [Frequency]

WEARABLE DATA SUMMARY

Average Resting Heart Rate: [Value] bpm

Average Sleep Duration: [Value] hours

Average HRV: [Value] ms

Steps per Day: [Value]

RECENT LAB RESULTS

[Test Name]: [Value] [Units] [Date]

[Test Name]: [Value] [Units] [Date]

2. **Save the file** and upload it along with any supporting documents when using AI tools

#### Method 3: Spreadsheet Approach (Advanced)

This method uses a structured spreadsheet that can be easily updated over time.

1. **Create an Excel or Google Sheets document** with separate tabs for the following:
    - Personal information
    - Genetic variants
    - Medications & supplements
    - Wearable data trends
    - Lab results history
2. **Format the genetic data** in a table with the following columns:
    - Gene
    - Variant (RS number if available)

- Your result
- Potential significance

3. **Save as CSV** file when needed for AI analysis

### Specialized Section: Using Pharmacogenomic Results with AI

Pharmacogenomic testing results are particularly valuable for medication analysis. Here's how to prepare this information for AI tools:

#### Step 1: Organize Your Medication Information

Create a spreadsheet or document with these columns:

- Medication
- Dosage
- Frequency
- Purpose
- Side effects experienced
- Start date

Include all prescription medications, over-the-counter drugs, and supplements.

#### Step 2: Extract Key Pharmacogenomic Data

From your pharmacogenomic test results, identify and list the following:

1. **Core metabolism genes** (focus on these critical enzymes)
    - *CYP2D6* (metabolizes ~25% of common drugs)
    - *CYP2C19* (processes antidepressants, antiplatelet drugs)
    - *CYP2C9* (affects warfarin, NSAIDs)

- *CYP3A4/CYP3A5* (metabolizes ~50% of medications)
- *VKORC1* (affects blood thinners)
- *SLCO1B1* (impacts statin metabolism)

2. **Your metabolizer status** for each gene
   - Ultrarapid metabolizer (UM)
   - Normal/extensive metabolizer (NM/EM)
   - Intermediate metabolizer (IM)
   - Poor metabolizer (PM)

### Step 3: Create a Simplified Report for AI

Format a document that clearly shows:

PHARMACOGENOMIC PROFILE

CYP2D6: [Your result, e.g., *1/*4] - [Metabolizer status, e.g., intermediate metabolizer]

Medications affected: [List from your test report]

CYP2C19: [Your result] - [Metabolizer status]

Medications affected: [List from your test report]

CURRENT MEDICATIONS AND SUPPLEMENTS

[Complete list as prepared in Step 1]

### Step 4: Specific Questions for AI Analysis

When uploading this information to an AI tool, consider asking the following:

1. "Based on my CYP2D6 status as an [X] metabolizer, are any of my current medications potentially problematic?"

2. "Are there any concerning interactions between my medications considering my pharmacogenomic profile?"
3. "Given my genetic results, what medication options might be better for [specific condition] if I need treatment in the future?"

### Prompting Tips for Better AI Analysis

When working with AI tools to analyze your combined health data, use these prompting strategies:

1. **Ask specific questions** rather than general ones
   - Good: "Based on my *MTHFR* variant and my wearable data showing poor sleep, what dietary adjustments might help?"
   - Less effective: "What do my genetics mean for my health?"
2. **Request prioritized insights**
   - "Please identify the top three actions I could take based on both my genetic and wearable data."
3. **Seek connections between data types**
   - "How might my *CYP2D6* status relate to the HRV patterns shown in my wearable data?"
4. **Ask for explanations in plain language**
   - "Please explain what my pharmacogenomic results mean for my medication choices in simple terms."

### Privacy and Security Considerations

When sharing health data with AI tools, take these precautions:

1. **Use trusted platforms** with clear privacy policies
2. **Consider anonymizing** your data by doing the following:
   - Remove your name and birthdate
   - Use initials or a pseudonym
   - Adjust your age to an age range (e.g., 40–45 instead of exact age)
3. **Use local AI tools** when possible, which process data on your device rather than sending it to external servers
4. **Check retention policies** to understand how long the AI service keeps your data

### Keeping Your Combined Health Data Updated

For ongoing health monitoring, do the following:

1. **Set a regular schedule** (monthly or quarterly) to update your health profile with the following:
   - New lab results
   - Medication changes
   - Updated wearable data summaries
2. **Track changes over time** by dating each update to your file or creating new versions
3. **Note correlations** you observe between different data types, such as the following:
   - Changes in sleep patterns when starting new supplements
   - Heart rate variations with medication adjustments
   - Energy levels in relation to specific biomarkers

By following these steps, you'll create a comprehensive health profile that allows AI tools to provide more personalized, meaningful insights that account for your unique genetic makeup alongside your day-to-day health metrics.

APPENDIX D

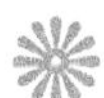

# GETTING DATA FROM YOUR SMART SCALES (E.G., WITHINGS BODY+, FITBIT ARIA)

Smart scales are valuable tools for tracking weight and body composition over time. The export methods described below work with current models from major manufacturers, but as technology advances, these steps might change. For the most current method specific to your device, try asking an AI assistant: "I have a [your scale brand and model]. What's the current method to export my weight and body composition data so I can analyze trends or share them with my doctor?" This approach ensures you'll always have instructions that work with the latest apps and features for your specific scale.

Smart scales are your daily health sidekick, tracking weight and body fat with ease. Here's how to collect that data, download it to your phone, analyze it with an AI like Grok 3, and turn the results into action. Whether you're on iPhone or Android, this guide's got you covered.

### Why Smart Scales Are a Big Deal

- **Rank:** Number two in my healthcare data lineup—right behind wearables.
- **Why It's Great:** Daily weight and body fat percentage show trends—a 10-pound gain over a year or creeping fat percentage can flag risks like diabetes, heart disease, or muscle loss (sarcopenia). They're more frequent than lab tests and sharper than occasional checkups. For a 62-year-old—or anyone—these tie straight to heart, metabolic, and joint health.
- **Quick Tip:** Weigh every morning, naked, after peeing—it's your simplest health snapshot.

### Do Smart Scales Download to Phone Apps?

Yes, the most common smart scales—like Withings Body+, Fitbit Aria, Eufy Smart Scale, Renpho, Wyze Scale, and Garmin Index—sync data to a phone app via Bluetooth or Wi-Fi. That's their superpower: automatic tracking directly to your device. The steps below work for these top players.

### Does Phone Type Matter?

Sort of. The process is the same whether you're on iOS (iPhone) or Android, but where the data goes differs.

- **iOS:** Syncs to Apple Health, then exports from there
- **Android:** Syncs to Google Fit, then exports from there

Some scales (e.g., Fitbit Aria) lean toward one ecosystem (Fitbit app, owned by Google), but most play nice with both via their own apps. Your phone type shapes the export path, not the collection.

### Step 1: Collecting the Data

Get consistent, reliable numbers—here's how:

- **When:** Every morning, post-bathroom, naked (no clothes to mess with the scale), which cuts out variables related to food, water, and fabric
- **What:** Step on—your scale grabs the following:
  - **Weight:** Tracks overall shifts—up, down, or steady
  - **Body Fat Percent:** Shows fat versus muscle—vital for metabolism and strength
- **How:** Set up your scale with its app
  - Pair it (Bluetooth/Wi-Fi) via Withings Health Mate, Fitbit, or similar
  - Input age, height, sex for accurate fat percentage
  - Weigh daily—it syncs to the app automatically
- **Why It Matters:** Daily data catches sneaky changes—like fluid buildup or fat gain—linked to heart strain or diabetes risk

### Step 2: Downloading the Data

Your scale's app sends data to your phone. Here's how to get it into Excel:

#### For iOS Users (iPhone)

- **Sync to Apple Health**
  - Open your scale's app (e.g., **Withings Health Mate, Fitbit**)
  - Go to **Settings > Apple Health** > Enable "Weight" and "Body Fat"

- **Export**
  - Open **Health app** > **Sources** > Your scale > **Export All Health Data** (XML)
  - Convert to CSV file with "Health Export" or "QS Access" (App Store)
  - Open in Excel, save as .xlsx

### For Android Users

- **Sync to Google Fit**
  - Open your scale's app (e.g., **Withings Health Mate**, **Fitbit**)
  - Go to **Settings > Google Fit** > Enable "Weight" and "Body Fat"
- **Export**
  - Visit **takeout.google.com** > Select "Fit" > Export as CSV file
  - Open in Excel, save as .xlsx
- **To AI**
  - **Grok 3:** Copy-paste 1–2 years of data into a query (e.g., "Here's my daily weight...")
  - **Other AIs:** Upload .xlsx/CSV file via "Attach File"

### Step 3: Directing the AI to Analyze

Tell the AI what to do. Keep it tight for clear insights.

- **Prompt:** "Analyze my smart scale data from [date range, up to 1–2 years]. Track weight and body fat percentage trends. Tie spikes or drops to specific times and suggest two or three practical steps to stabilize or improve—like diet or exercise tweaks"

- **Why It Works:** Daily weigh-ins give AI tons to chew on—365+ data points yearly—to spot stuff like "Your weight spiked after late-night snacks" and link it to health risks

### Step 4: What to Do with the Results

AI hands you insights. Here's how to use them with daily data:

- If Weight Climbs (e.g., 10 pounds in a year)
  - **AI Might Say:** "Your weight rose with less activity—add 20-min walks"
  - **You Do:** Move more (walks, stairs), cut snacks—small changes stick
  - **Why:** Gradual gains hint at obesity or fluid issues—potential heart and diabetes markers
- **If Body Fat Percentage Jumps (e.g., 5% in 6 months)**
  - **AI Might Say:** "Fat percent up, sleep down—aim for 7+ hours"
  - **You Do:** Sleep better, lift weights—muscle fights fat
  - **Why:** Fat over muscle (sarcopenia) slows metabolism, stresses joints—big at age 62
- **If Stable but Risky (e.g., BMI 32, fat percentage 35%)**
  - **AI Might Say:** "Steady but high—cut carbs, build muscle"
  - **You Do:** Drop sugar, lift light weights—long-game health win
  - **Why:** High baselines still spell CVD trouble—daily tracking keeps the risk front and center.

- **Bonus:** Pair with wearables or blood pressure data (Appendices A/B) for the full story (e.g., "Weight up + blood pressure rising = cut stress")

### Practical Use Wrap-Up

- **For You:** AI connects weight jumps to life (e.g., "Fat percent rose with fewer steps—move more"), which enables you to see the why and how
- **For a 62-Year-Old:** Daily data spot risks early—obesity, heart strain, muscle fade—letting you tweak habits before bigger issues hit
- **Patient Pitch:** "Step on daily—it's your easiest health measurement, so let AI make it a plan"

APPENDIX E

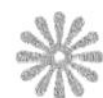

# USING AI TO FIND, ADMINISTER, AND SCORE MENTAL HEALTH SCREENING TOOLS

This appendix provides step-by-step guidance on using AI to help access, complete, and interpret validated mental health screening instruments with privacy in mind.

## Finding the Right Screening Tool Based on Wearable Data

Your wearable device may show patterns that suggest specific mental health concerns. Here's how to identify which screening tool might be most relevant:

### For Sleep Disturbances Detected by Your Wearable

- **Insomnia** (difficulty falling or staying asleep): Consider the PHQ-9 for depression screening, as persistent insomnia is present in 80–85% of depression cases
- **Hypersomnia** (excessive sleeping): The PHQ-9 is also appropriate, as unusual increases in sleep duration can signal depression

- **Irregular Sleep Patterns**: Consider both PHQ-9 and GAD-7, as disrupted sleep can indicate either depression or anxiety

### For Heart Rate and Activity Anomalies

- **Elevated Resting Heart Rate:** The GAD-7 can help screen for anxiety, which often manifests as increased heart rate
- **Decreased Daily Activity:** The PHQ-9 might be appropriate, as reduced movement can correlate with depression
- **High Heart Rate Variability During Rest Periods:** Consider the PCL-5 for PTSD, which can cause physiological hyperarousal

### For Irregular Eating or Weight Changes

- **Rapid Weight Loss or Gain:** The PHQ-9 can help screen for depression, which often affects appetite
- **Meal Skipping Patterns:** Consider screening tools for eating disorders such as the Eating Attitudes Test (EAT-26)

## Step-by-Step Guide to Using AI for Mental Health Screening

### Step 1: Request Information About Appropriate Tools

With a natural language AI assistant, use queries like the following:

- "Based on my wearable data showing [specific pattern], which mental health screening tool would be most appropriate?"

- "What validated questionnaire would help assess symptoms of [concern]?"
- "Can you explain what the PHQ-9 measures and how it works?"

**Privacy Tip:** When describing your symptoms or concerns to AI, avoid including personally identifiable information. Use general descriptions rather than specific dates, names, or locations.

### Step 2: Accessing the Screening Tool

Most validated screening tools are publicly available but may have copyright protections. Here's how to find them:

1. **Using AI Guidance:** Ask: "Where can I find the official version of [screening tool]?"
2. **Direct Sources:** Visit these reliable websites that host official versions
   - PHQ-9: https://www.phqscreeners.com/ (free for clinical and research use)
   - GAD-7: https://www.phqscreeners.com/ (same site as PHQ-9)
   - AUDIT: Available through the World Health Organization website
   - PCL-5: Available through the National Center for PTSD website
   - MDQ: Available through various mental health organizations
3. **Privacy-Focused Completion:** For maximum privacy, download the PDF version when available rather than completing it online

**Privacy Tip:** Use a private/incognito browsing window when accessing these tools to minimize tracking. Some browsers like Firefox Focus or Brave offer enhanced privacy features.

### Step 3: Scoring and Interpretation

After completing the assessment, you can use AI to help score and interpret the results.

1. **For Scoring Assistance:** Tell the AI: "I answered [list your responses] on the PHQ-9. How is this scored?"
2. **For Interpretation:** Ask: "What does a score of [X] on the [screening tool] suggest?"
3. **For Context:** Request: "How common is a score of [X] on the [screening tool]?"

**Privacy Tip:** When sharing your responses with AI, you don't need to explain why you answered a certain way—just provide the numerical responses (e.g., "I answered 2,1,3,2,1,0,2,1,1 on the PHQ-9").

### Step 4: Next Steps Based on Results

AI can help you understand appropriate follow-up actions.

1. **For Moderate Scores:** Ask: "What self-care strategies might help with a [moderate] score on [screening tool]?"
2. **For Higher Scores:** Request: "When should someone with a score of [X] on the [screening tool] seek professional help?"
3. **For Resource Guidance:** Enquire: "What types of mental health professionals treat [condition]?"

**Privacy Tip:** If you're concerned about your results, consider using a secure telehealth platform to discuss them with a healthcare provider rather than storing this sensitive information in AI chat logs.

### Using Specialized Mental Health AI Applications

Several AI applications are designed for mental health support with stronger privacy protections:

1. **Woebot:** An evidence-based mental health chatbot that uses CBT techniques
   - Privacy benefit: Designed with healthcare privacy standards in mind
   - Access: Available as a mobile app (iOS/Android)
2. **Wysa:** AI chatbot combining CBT, dialectical behavior therapy (DBT), and meditation techniques.
   - Privacy benefit: Anonymous usage option available
   - Access: Available as a mobile app (iOS/Android)
3. **Youper:** AI-powered emotional health assistant
   - Privacy benefit: HIPAA-compliant
   - Access: Available as a mobile app (iOS/Android)

**Important Note:** While these specialized apps generally offer stronger privacy protections than general-purpose AI, always review their privacy policies carefully.

### When to Seek Human Help

AI tools should complement, not replace, professional care. Seek immediate professional help if you experience any of the following:

- Thoughts of harming yourself or others
- Inability to perform daily functions or self-care
- Severe symptoms that significantly impair your quality of life
- Psychotic symptoms (hallucinations or delusions)

In these situations, contact your healthcare provider, visit an emergency room, or call the National Suicide Prevention Lifeline (988) immediately.

Remember that screening tools and AI assistance are starting points for understanding your mental health, not diagnostic tools. A healthcare professional should always make formal diagnoses and treatment recommendations.

APPENDIX F

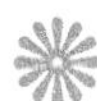

# HEALTH APPS

| App Name | Description | Access Method |
|---|---|---|
| Ada Health | An AI-driven symptom checker and health guide that provides personalized health insights, preventive advice, and care options based on user symptoms and medical guidelines. | Available on iOS and Android app stores; search for "Ada Health" or visit ada.com. |
| AirNow | A smart air quality app that uses AI to predict local air quality, helping users plan activities to avoid pollution-related lung risks. | Available on iOS and Android app stores; search for "AirNow" or visit airnow.gov. |
| AirThings Wave | A smart device for continuous radon level monitoring, sending alerts to your phone when levels are high. | Purchase device from airthings.com; app available on iOS and Android app stores as "AirThings." |

| App Name | Description | Access Method |
|---|---|---|
| AllTrails | Recommends walking routes based on user preferences for terrain, greenery, or quiet areas, supporting stress reduction and physical activity. | Available on iOS and Android app stores; search for "AllTrails" or visit alltrails.com. |
| Athlytic | A data-driven fitness app that uses AI to analyze sleep, activity, and recovery trends from connected health devices, offering actionable insights. | Available on iOS app store; search for "Athlytic." Subscription: $3/month. |
| Aysa | Uses AI to assist in dermatological diagnoses by analyzing user-uploaded photos, providing preliminary insights into skin conditions. | Available on iOS and Android app stores; search for "Aysa" or visit aysaapp.com. |
| Bite AI | Analyzes eating behavior (speed, bite size, meal duration) using phone camera data to promote mindful eating and reduce overconsumption. | Available on iOS and Android app stores; search for "Bite AI." |
| Brain.fm | Creates AI-generated sounds to guide brain waves into optimal frequencies for napping or relaxation. | Available on iOS and Android app stores; search for "Brain.fm" or visit brain.fm. |
| Breezometer | Uses AI to predict local air quality, helping users avoid pollution-related lung risks by suggesting safe times for outdoor activities. | Available on iOS and Android app stores; search for "Breezometer" or visit breezometer.com. |

| App Name | Description | Access Method |
|---|---|---|
| Buoy | An AI-powered symptom checker that provides possible diagnoses, educational materials, and next steps based on user symptoms. | Available on iOS and Android app stores; search for "Buoy Health" or visit buoyhealth.com. |
| Cardiogram | Detects irregular heart rhythms with 97% accuracy using wearable data, aiding in heart health monitoring. | Available on iOS and Android app stores; search for "Cardiogram." Subscription: $0–14.99/month. |
| Carrot | A fitness app using AI to provide motivational support with humorous commentary, rewards, and adaptive workouts. | Available on iOS and Android app stores; search for "Carrot Fit." |
| Community Health AI | Connects users with culturally tailored online support groups for smoking cessation and health management. | Availability varies; search for "Community Health AI" on iOS/Android app stores or community health platforms. |
| Cronometer | Tracks nutrient intake from food and supplements, offering free and premium versions for detailed dietary analysis. | Available on iOS and Android app stores; search for "Cronometer" or visit cronometer.com. Subscription: Free, with premium options ($6/month). |

| App Name | Description | Access Method |
|---|---|---|
| CultureQuit | Provides culturally tailored advice for smoking cessation, particularly for Black American menthol cigarette users, increasing quit rates by 41%. | Available on iOS and Android app stores; search for "CultureQuit." |
| Daylio | Connects mood entries with activities to identify which forms of play boost mental state, supporting mental health. | Available on iOS and Android app stores; search for "Daylio" or visit daylio.net. |
| DeepCare AI | An AI-powered assistant for medical insights, symptom analysis, and doctor appointment booking. | Available on iOS and Android app stores; search for "DeepCare AI" or visit lablab.ai for similar platforms. |
| EasyQuit | Tracks money saved, time since last cigarette, and cravings, using gamified features for smoking cessation. | Available on iOS and Android app stores; search for "EasyQuit." |
| Eight Sleep Pod | Adjusts bed temperature to optimize sleep based on user patterns, enhancing sleep quality. | Purchase device from eightsleep.com; app available on iOS and Android app stores as "Eight Sleep." |
| Elicit AI | Summarizes medical research in plain language, helping users understand complex studies. | Available at elicit.org; access via web browser. |

| App Name | Description | Access Method |
|---|---|---|
| Fast Habit | Suggests optimal eating windows for intermittent fasting based on user activity and energy levels. | Available on iOS and Android app stores; search for "Fast Habit." |
| Fitbod | Provides AI-driven personalized workout recommendations based on user progress and goals. | Available on iOS and Android app stores; search for "Fitbod" or visit fitbod.me. |
| Fooducate | Uses AI to scan barcodes and warn about unhealthy ingredients, added sugars, and false health claims. | Available on iOS and Android app stores; search for "Fooducate" or visit fooducate.com. |
| Future | Offers AI-driven personalized workout recommendations, adapting to user progress and goals. | Available on iOS and Android app stores; search for "Future" or visit future.co. |
| GI Genius | Works with doctors during colonoscopies to highlight polyps, increasing detection by 10–15%. | Available through medical facilities using Medtronic's GI Genius system; ask your provider. |
| Google Fit | Centralizes health data (steps, heart rate, sleep) and integrates with wearables for comprehensive tracking. | Preinstalled on Android devices or available on iOS/Android app stores; search for "Google Fit." |
| H1 | Connects healthcare professionals for networking and knowledge exchange using AI. | Available at h1.co; access via web browser or contact for app availability. |

| App Name | Description | Access Method |
|---|---|---|
| Headspace | Offers AI-supported meditation and stress reduction exercises to improve mental health. | Available on iOS and Android app stores; search for "Headspace" or visit headspace.com. |
| Heads Up Health | Integrates medical records, lab results, wearable data, and nutrition tracking into comprehensive dashboards. | Available on iOS and Android app stores; search for "Heads Up Health" or visit headsuphealth.com. |
| HealthyYou Colon | Provides personalized screening reminders for colon cancer based on user risk factors. | Available on iOS and Android app stores; search for "HealthyYou Colon." |
| HeartWatch | Provides detailed insights into heart rate patterns, enhancing cardiovascular monitoring. | Available on iOS app store; search for "HeartWatch." Cost: $4.99. |
| Human Dx | Assists healthcare professionals with diagnoses across specialties, supporting initial assessments. | Available at humandx.org; access via web browser or app stores as "Human Dx." |
| Hydration AI | Suggests optimal times for hydration based on user activity and environmental data. | Available through Gatorade's app; search for "Gatorade" on iOS/Android app stores. |
| iHairium | Uses AI computer vision to analyze hair and scalp health from photos, suggesting treatments for hair loss. | Available on iOS and Android app stores; search for "iHairium." |

| App Name | Description | Access Method |
|---|---|---|
| JourneyAI | Checks product ingredients against research to provide evidence-based nutrition advice. | Availability varies; search for "JourneyAI" on iOS/ Android app stores or health platforms. |
| Kareo | Streamlines medical billing processes using AI, reducing administrative burdens for providers. | Available at kareo.com; access via web browser or contact for app availability. |
| Klara | Streamlines administrative tasks and patient communication for healthcare providers, automating scheduling and reminders. | Available on iOS and Android app stores; search for "Klara" or visit klara.com. |
| Kwit | Tracks smoking cessation progress, including money saved and cravings, using gamified milestones. | Available on iOS and Android app stores; search for "Kwit." |
| Lark Health | Coaches blood pressure management and provides personalized health advice using AI. | Available on iOS and Android app stores; search for "Lark" or visit lark.com. Subscription: $20/ month. |
| Levels | Pairs with continuous glucose monitors to visualize blood sugar responses to foods, offering personalized nutrition advice. | Available on iOS and Android app stores; search for "Levels" or visit levelshealth.com. |

| App Name | Description | Access Method |
|---|---|---|
| LIFE Fasting Tracker | Supports intermittent fasting by predicting slip risks and offering support. | Available on iOS and Android app stores; search for "LIFE Fasting Tracker." |
| Lumen | You breathe into a device that analyzes your breath to see if your body is burning carbs or fat for energy right now. Once you know which fuel you're using, you can time your meals better—eating carbs when your body needs quick energy, or fasting when it's efficiently burning fat. | Purchase device from lumen.me; app available on iOS and Android app stores as "Lumen." |
| Lumosity | Offers cognitive assessment and brain training exercises to detect early cognitive changes. | Available on iOS and Android app stores; search for "Lumosity" or visit lumosity.com. |
| Medisafe | A medication management tool with AI-driven interaction alerts and reminders. | Available on iOS and Android app stores; search for "Medisafe" or visit medisafe.com. |
| MedWise | Provides medication risk scores and interaction checks using AI. | Available at medwise.com; access via web browser or contact for app availability. |
| Meetup | Suggests local playful social activities to boost mental health and reduce stress. | Available on iOS and Android app stores; search for "Meetup" or visit meetup.com. |

| App Name | Description | Access Method |
|---|---|---|
| Metric Health | Uses wearable data to predict metabolic problems before standard tests, aiding early intervention. | Availability varies; search for "MetricHealth" on iOS/ Android app stores or health platforms. |
| Mindful Meal | Uses AI to study food-emotion connections, supporting mindful eating for weight management. | Available on iOS and Android app stores; search for "Mindful Meal." |
| MindHaven | An AI-powered mental health companion offering emotional support, mindfulness, and journaling. | Available on iOS and Android app stores; search for "MindHaven" or visit lablab.ai. |
| Mindstrong | Analyzes phone usage patterns to detect cognitive changes or stress, supporting mental health monitoring. | Availability varies; search for "Mindstrong" on iOS/ Android app stores or mental health platforms. |
| Motion | Identifies meetings suitable for walking to promote physical activity and stress reduction. | Available on iOS and Android app stores; search for "Motion." |
| MyFitnessPal | Tracks food intake and nutrients, offering free basic nutrient tracking for dietary management. | Available on iOS and Android app stores; search for "MyFitnessPal" or visit myfitnesspal.com. |

| App Name | Description | Access Method |
|---|---|---|
| MyTherapy | Manages medication schedules and tracks symptoms with AI-driven reminders. | Available on iOS and Android app stores; search for "MyTherapy" or visit mytherapyapp.com. |
| Nanox | Integrates AI into medical imaging for cost-effective diagnostic solutions. | Available through medical facilities; visit nanox.vision for provider information. |
| NapBot | Suggests ideal nap times based on body rhythm dips, optimizing rest. | Available on iOS and Android app stores; search for "NapBot." |
| NutriCare Agents | Provides personalized meal plans using AI, integrating local food data for health and sustainability. | Available on iOS and Android app stores; search for "NutriCare Agents" or visit lablab.ai. |
| Oblique Strategies | Generates creative prompts tailored to user interests for mental health and creativity. | Available on iOS and Android app stores; search for "Oblique Strategies." |
| Playtime AI | Suggests playful activities matched to user personality to boost mental health. | Availability varies; search for "Playtime AI" on iOS/Android app stores or mental health platforms. |
| Propeller | Tracks breathing and air quality data to manage asthma, providing alerts for triggers. | Available on iOS and Android app stores; search for "Propeller" or visit propellerhealth.com. |

| App Name | Description | Access Method |
|---|---|---|
| PurpleAir | Uses AI to predict local air quality, helping users avoid pollution-related lung risks. | Available on iOS and Android app stores; search for "PurpleAir" or visit purpleair.com. |
| Pzizz | Analyzes nap data to recommend optimal nap durations (20 or 90 minutes) for rest. | Available on iOS and Android app stores; search for "Pzizz" or visit pzizz.com. |
| quitSTART | A free CDC app for smoking cessation, offering tips, challenges, and craving trackers. | Available on iOS and Android app stores; search for "quitSTART" or visit cdc.gov. |
| QuitGenius | Analyzes wearable data to support smoking cessation, increasing quit rates by 36%. | Available on iOS and Android app stores; search for "QuitGenius" or visit quitgenius.com. |
| QuitSure | Uses mindfulness and therapy to reduce withdrawal symptoms in smoking cessation. | Available on iOS and Android app stores; search for "QuitSure." |
| Recovery Record | Uses AI to study food-emotion connections, offering privacy mode for eating disorder management. | Available on iOS and Android app stores; search for "Recovery Record" or visit recoveryrecord.com. |
| Reflex | Uses AI pose estimation to assess and track shoulder mobility recovery at home. | Available on iOS and Android app stores; search for "Reflex." |

| App Name | Description | Access Method |
|---|---|---|
| ResearchAssistant | Monitors new medical publications and alerts users to relevant studies. | Availability varies; search for "ResearchAssistant" on iOS/Android app stores or research platforms. |
| Rise Science | Times morning light exposure based on sleep data and sunrise times to improve mood and sleep. | Available on iOS and Android app stores; search for "Rise: Sleep Tracker" or visit risescience.com. |
| SaunaSpace | Tailors sauna sessions to user goals, monitoring heart rate for safety. | Purchase device from saunaspace.com; app available on iOS and Android app stores as "SaunaSpace." |
| Scite | Summarizes medical research in plain language, aiding patient understanding. | Available at scite.ai; access via web browser as "Scite." |
| Sleep Cycle | Analyzes sleep quality and wakes users during light sleep phases for better rest. | Available on iOS and Android app stores; search for "Sleep Cycle" or visit sleepcycle.com. Subscription: $39.99/year. |
| Sleep.ai | Tracks sleep quality and mood improvements from lifestyle changes like morning light exposure. | Available on iOS and Android app stores; search for "Sleep.ai." |

| App Name | Description | Access Method |
|---|---|---|
| SleepSpace | Identifies behaviors impacting sleep quality, offering tailored suggestions. | Available on iOS and Android app stores; search for "SleepSpace" or visit sleepspace.com. |
| Spire Stone | Detects breathing patterns linked to stress, offering early relaxation alerts. | Purchase device from spirehealth.com; app available on iOS and Android app stores as "Spire." |
| Strava | Recommends walking routes based on user preferences, supporting physical activity. | Available on iOS and Android app stores; search for "Strava" or visit strava.com. |
| Trauma Recovery | Offers AI-powered adverse childhood experiences survey for trauma-related weight management. | Available on iOS and Android app stores; search for "Trauma Recovery." |
| WaterMinder | Calculates hydration needs based on weight, activity, and temperature, sending reminders. | Available on iOS and Android app stores; search for "WaterMinder" or visit waterminder.com. |
| Wellory | Tracks how breathing exercises impact stress signals, supporting relaxation. | Available on iOS and Android app stores; search for "Wellory." |
| WHOOP | Provides advanced sleep and recovery analysis using HRV, respiratory rate, and sleep architecture. | Purchase device from whoop.com; app available on iOS and Android app stores as "WHOOP." Subscription: $30/month. |

| App Name | Description | Access Method |
|---|---|---|
| Withings Health Mate | Detects heart rate and blood pressure changes signaling dehydration or health issues. | Available on iOS and Android app stores; search for "Withings Health Mate" or visit withings.com. |
| Withings Sleep Analyzer | Examines sleep structure to optimize mental and physical recovery. | Purchase device from withings.com; app available on iOS and Android app stores as "Withings Health Mate." |
| Wysa | Analyzes user conversations and emotions to provide personalized mental health support and coping strategies. | Available on iOS and Android app stores; search for "Wysa" or visit wysa.io. Subscription: Free, with premium options. |
| Youper | Tracks mood and provides personalized mental health insights with a free trial. | Available on iOS and Android app stores; search for "Youper" or visit youper.ai. |
| Zero | Suggests fasting protocols (e.g., 16:8, 5:2) based on user health and goals, tracking progress. | Available on iOS and Android app stores; search for "Zero" or visit zeroapp.io. |

# REFERENCES

This list includes all books, articles, and studies mentioned in the chapters, plus additional references that support the topics discussed.

## Introduction


1. American Medical Association. (2024). *Augmented intelligence development, deployment, and use in health care* [Board Report]. https://www.ama-assn.org/system/files/ama-ai-principles.pdf

2. American Thyroid Association. (2020). *General information/press room.* https://www.thyroid.org/media-main/press-room/

3. Asan, O., Bayrak, A. E., & Choudhury, A. (2020). Artificial intelligence and human trust in healthcare: Focus on clinicians. *Journal of Medical Internet Research, 22*(6), Article e15154. https://doi.org/10.2196/15154

4. Attia, Z. I., Noseworthy, P. A., Lopez-Jimenez, F., Asirvatham, S. J., Deshmukh, A. J., Gersh, B. J., ... & Friedman, P. A. (2019). An artificial intelligence-enabled ECG algorithm for the identification of patients with atrial fibrillation during sinus rhythm: a retrospective analysis of outcome prediction. *The Lancet, 394*(10201), 861–867. https://doi.org/10.1016/S0140-6736(19)31721-0

5. Borchert, R. J., Azevedo, T., Badhwar, A., Bernal, J., Betts, M., Bruffaerts, R., Burkhart, M. C., Dewachter, I., Gellersen, H. M., Low, A., Lourida, I., Machado, L., Madan, C. R., Malpetti, M., Mejia, J., Michopoulou, S., Muñoz-Neira, C., Pepys, J., Peres, M., ... Rittman, T. (2023). Artificial intelligence for diagnostic and prognostic neuroimaging in dementia: A systematic review. *Alzheimer's & Dementia, 19(*12), 5885–5904. https://doi.org/10.1002/alz.13412

6. Chen, J. H., & Asch, S. M. (2017). Machine learning and prediction in medicine–Beyond the peak of inflated expectations. *New England Journal of Medicine, 376*(26), 2507–2509. https://doi.org/10.1056/NEJMp1702071

7. Davenport, T. H., & Kalakota, R. (2019). The potential for artificial intelligence in healthcare. *Future Healthcare Journal*, *6*(2), 94–98. https://doi.org/10.7861/futurehosp.6-2-94

8. Ellahham, S. (2020). Artificial intelligence: The future for diabetes care. *The American Journal of Medicine, 133*(8), 895–900. https://doi.org/10.1016/j.amjmed.2020.03.033

9. Elwyn, G., Frosch, D., Thomson, R., Joseph-Williams, N., Lloyd, A., Kinnersley, P., Cording, E., Tomson, D., Dodd, C., Rollnick, S., Edwards, A., & Barry, M. (2012). Shared decision making: A model for clinical practice. *Journal of General Internal Medicine, 27*(10), 1361–1367. https://doi.org/10.1007/s11606-012-2077-6

10. Flores, L. E., Frontera, W. R., Andrasik, M. P., del Rio, C., Mondríguez-González, A., Price, S. A., Krantz, E. M.,

Pergam, S. A., & Silver, J. K. (2021). Assessment of the inclusion of racial/ethnic minority, female, and older individuals in vaccine clinical trials. *JAMA Network Open*, *4*(2), Article e2037640. https://doi.org/10.1001/jamanetworkopen.2020.37640

11. Fontanarosa, P. B., & Bauchner, H. (2018). Race, ancestry, and medical research. *JAMA*, *320*(15), 1539–1540. https://doi.org/10.1001/jama.2018.14438
12. Hosny, A., Parmar, C., Quackenbush, J., Schwartz, L. H., & Aerts, H. J. W. L. (2018). Artificial intelligence in radiology. *Nature Reviews Cancer*, *18*(8), 500–510. https://doi.org/10.1038/s41568-018-0016-5
13. Ioannidis, J. P. A., Powe, N. R., & Yancy, C. (2021). Recalibrating the use of race in medical research. *JAMA*, *325*(7), 623–624. https://doi.org/10.1001/jama.2021.0003
14. Kaiser Family Foundation & The Undefeated. (2020, October 13). *KFF/The Undefeated survey on race and health*. https://www.kff.org/report-section/kff-the-undefeated-survey-on-race-and-health-main-findings/
15. Katz, U., Cohen, E., Shachar, E., Somer, J., Fink, A., Morse, E., Shreiber, B., & Wolf, I. (2024). GPT versus resident physicians—A benchmark based on official board scores. *NEJM AI*, *1*(4), Article AIdbp2300192. https://doi.org/10.1056/AIdbp2300192
16. Liu, M., Okuhara, T., Chang, X., Shirabe, R., Nishiie, Y., Okada, H., & Kiuchi, T. (2024). Performance of ChatGPT across different versions in medical licensing examinations worldwide: Systematic review and meta-analysis. *Journal of Medical Internet Research*, *26*, Article e60807. https://doi.org/10.2196/60807

17. Majumder, M. A., Guerrini, C. J., & McGuire, A. L. (2021). Direct-to-consumer genetic testing: Value and risk. *Annual Review of Medicine, 72*, 151–166. https://doi.org/10.1146/annurev-med-070119-114727

18. McCambridge, J., Witton, J., & Elbourne, D. R. (2014). Systematic review of the Hawthorne effect: New concepts are needed to study research participation effects. *Journal of Clinical Epidemiology, 67*(3), 267–277. https://doi.org/10.1016/j.jclinepi.2013.08.015

19. Obermeyer, Z., Powers, B., Vogeli, C., & Mullainathan, S. (2019). Dissecting racial bias in an algorithm used to manage the health of populations. *Science, 366*(6464), 447–453. https://doi.org/10.1126/science.aax2342

20. Oh, S. S., Galanter, J., Thakur, N., Pino-Yanes, M., Barcelo, N. E., White, M. J., de Bruin, D. M., Greenblatt, R. M., Bibbins-Domingo, K., Wu, A. H. B., Borrell, L. N., Gunter, C., Powe, N. R., & Burchard, E. G. (2015). Diversity in clinical and biomedical research: A promise yet to be fulfilled. *PLOS Medicine, 12*(12), Article e1001918. https://doi.org/10.1371/journal.pmed.1001918

21. Price, W. N., & Cohen, I. G. (2019). Privacy in the age of medical big data. *Nature Medicine, 25*(1), 37–43. https://doi.org/10.1038/s41591-018-0272-7

22. Rajpurkar, P., Chen, E., Banerjee, O., & Topol, E. J. (2022). AI in health and medicine. *Nature Medicine, 28*(1), 31–38. https://doi.org/10.1038/s41591-021-01614-0

23. Reddy, S., Fox, J., & Purohit, M. P. (2019). Artificial intelligence-enabled healthcare delivery. *Journal of the Royal Society of Medicine, 112*(1), 22–28. https://doi.org/10.1177/0141076818815510

24. Reddy, S., Allan, S., Coghlan, S., & Cooper, P. (2020). A governance model for the application of AI in health care. *Journal of the American Medical Informatics Association, 27*(3), 491–497. https://doi.org/10.1093/jamia/ocz192

25. Rubin, E. J. (2021). Striving for diversity in research studies. *New England Journal of Medicine, 385*(15), 1429–1430. https://doi.org/10.1056/NEJMe2114651

26. Scheibner, J., Raisaro, J. L., Troncoso-Pastoriza, J. R., Ienca, M., Fellay, J., Vayena, E., & Hubaux, J. P. (2021). Revolutionizing medical data sharing using advanced privacy-enhancing technologies: Technical, legal, and ethical synthesis. *Journal of Medical Internet Research, 23*(2), Article e25120. https://doi.org/10.2196/25120

27. Schork, N.J. (2019). Artificial intelligence and personalized medicine. In Von Hoff, D., & Han, H. (Eds.), *Precision Medicine in Cancer Therapy* (pp 265–283). Springer. https://doi.org/10.1007/978-3-030-16391-4_11

28. Shen, Y., Heacock, L., Elias, J., Hentel, K. D., Reig, B., Shih, G., & Moy, L. (2023). ChatGPT and other large language models are double-edged swords. *Radiology, 307*(2), e230163. https://doi.org/10.1148/radiol.230163

29. Topol, E. J. (2019). *Deep medicine: How artificial intelligence can make healthcare human again*. Basic Books.

30. Topol E. J. (2019). High-performance medicine: the convergence of human and artificial intelligence. *Nature Medicine, 25*(1), 44–56. https://doi.org/10.1038/s41591-018-0300-7

31. U.S. Department of Health and Human Services. (2021). *2021 report to Congress on breaches of unsecured*

*protected health information.* https://www.hhs.gov/sites/default/files/breach-report-to-congress-2021.pdf

32. Zeevi, D., Korem, T., Zmora, N., Israeli, D., Rothschild, D., Weinberger, A., Ben-Yacov, O., Lador, D., Avnit-Sagi, T., Lotan-Pompan, M., Suez, J., Mahdi, J. A., Matot, E., Malka, G., Kosower, N., Rein, M., Zilberman-Schapira, G., Dohnalová, L., Pevsner-Fischer, M., & Segal, E. (2015). Personalized nutrition by prediction of glycemic responses. *Cell, 163*(5), 1079–1094. https://doi.org/10.1016/j.cell.2015.11.001

## Part 1: Reading Your Body's Signals

### The Health Diary on Your Wrist

1. Arkenberg, C. (2021, July 30). *Wearables in health care: Current and future applications.* Deloitte Insights. https://www.deloitte.com/us/en/insights/industry/technology/wearable-technology-healthcare-data.html
2. Attia, Z. I., Noseworthy, P. A., Lopez-Jimenez, F., Asirvatham, S. J., Deshmukh, A. J., Gersh, B. J., Carter, R. E., Yao, X., Rabinstein, A. A., Erickson, B. J., Kapa, S., & Friedman, P. A. (2019). An artificial intelligence-enabled ECG algorithm for the identification of patients with atrial fibrillation during sinus rhythm: A retrospective analysis of outcome prediction. *The Lancet, 394*(10201), 861–867. https://doi.org/10.1016/S0140-6736(19)31721-0
3. Bayo-Monton, J. L., Martinez-Millana, A., Han, W., Fernandez-Llatas, C., Sun, Y., & Traver, V. (2018). Wearable sensors integrated with Internet of Things for advancing

eHealth care. *Sensors, 18*(6), Article 1851. https://doi.org/10.3390/s18061851

4. Colilla, S., Crow, A., Petkun, W., Singer, D. E., Simon, T., & Liu, X. (2013). Estimates of current and future incidence and prevalence of atrial fibrillation in the U.S. adult population. *American Journal of Cardiology, 112*(8), 1142–1147. https://doi.org/10.1016/j.amjcard.2013.05.063

5. Dobson, J., Whitley, R. J., Pocock, S., & Monto, A. S. (2015). Oseltamivir treatment for influenza in adults: A meta-analysis of randomised controlled trials. *The Lancet, 385*(9979), 1729–1737. https://doi.org/10.1016/S0140-6736(14)62449-1

6. Haghayegh, S., Khoshnevis, S., Smolensky, M. H., Diller, K. R., & Castriotta, R. J. (2019). Accuracy of wristband Fitbit models in assessing sleep: Systematic review and meta-analysis. *Journal of Medical Internet Research, 21*(11), Article e16273. https://doi.org/10.2196/16273

7. Hart, R. G., Pearce, L. A., & Aguilar, M. I. (2007). Meta-analysis: Antithrombotic therapy to prevent stroke in patients who have nonvalvular atrial fibrillation. *Annals of Internal Medicine, 146*(12), 857–867. https://doi.org/10.7326/0003-4819-146-12-200706190-00007

8. Hemilä, H., & Chalker, E. (2013). Vitamin C for preventing and treating the common cold. *Cochrane Database of Systematic Reviews, 2013*(1), Article CD000980. https://doi.org/10.1002/14651858.CD000980.pub4

9. Kositpantawong, N., Surasombatpattana, S., Siripaitoon, P., Kanchanasuwan, S., Hortiwakul, T.,

Charernmak, B., & Chusri, S. (2021). Outcomes of early oseltamivir treatment for hospitalized adult patients with community-acquired influenza pneumonia. *PLOS One, 16*(12), Article e0261411. https://doi.org/10.1371/journal.pone.0261411

10. Nelson, B. W., & Allen, N. B. (2019). Accuracy of consumer wearable heart rate measurement during an ecologically valid 24-hour period: Intraindividual validation study. *JMIR mHealth and uHealth, 8*(3), Article e10828. https://doi.org/10.2196/10828
11. Pew Research Center. (2021). *Mobile fact sheet.* https://www.pewresearch.org/internet/fact-sheet/mobile/
12. Rajkomar, A., Dean, J., & Kohane, I. (2019). Machine learning in medicine. *New England Journal of Medicine, 380*(14), 1347–1358. https://doi.org/10.1056/NEJMra1814259
13. Rock Health. (2024, August 5). *Put a ring on it: Understanding consumers' year-over-year wearable adoption patterns.* https://rockhealth.com/insights/put-a-ring-on-it-understanding-consumers-year-over-year-wearable-adoption-patterns/
14. Wolf, P. A., Abbott, R. D., & Kannel, W. B. (1991). Atrial fibrillation as an independent risk factor for stroke: The Framingham Study. *Stroke, 22*(8), 983–988. https://doi.org/10.1161/01.str.22.8.983

## AI Can Find Hidden Health Secrets in Your Genes

1. Allyse, M. A., Robinson, D. H., Ferber, M. J., & Sharp, R. R. (2018). Direct-to-consumer testing 2.0: emerging

models of direct-to-consumer genetic testing. *Mayo Clinic Proceedings*, *93*(1), 113–120. https://doi.org/10.1016/j.mayocp.2017.11.001

2. Bean, L. J. H., Scheuner, M. T., Murray, M. F., Biesecker, L. G., Green, R. C., Monaghan, K. G., Palomaki, G. E., Sharp, R. R., Trotter, T. L., Watson, M. S., Powell, C. M., & ACMG Board of Directors (2021). DNA-based screening and personal health: a points to consider statement for individuals and health-care providers from the American College of Medical Genetics and Genomics (ACMG). *Genetics in Medicine : Official Journal of the American College of Medical Genetics*, *23*(6), 979–988. https://doi.org/10.1038/s41436-020-01083-9

3. Daly, M. B., Pal, T., Maxwell, K. N., Churpek, J., Kohlmann, W., AlHilli, Z., Arun, B., Buys, S. S., Cheng, H., Domchek, S. M., Friedman, S., Giri, V. N., Goggins, M., Hagemann, A. R., Hendrix, A., Hutton, M. L., Karlan, B. Y., Kassem, N., Khan, S., ... Dwyer, M. A. (2023). NCCN guidelines insights: Genetic/familial high-risk assessment: Breast, ovarian, and pancreatic, version 2.2024. *Journal of the National Comprehensive Cancer Network*, *21*(10), 1000–1010. https://doi.org/10.6004/jnccn.2023.0051

4. Dias, R., & Torkamani, A. (2019). Artificial intelligence in clinical and genomic diagnostics. *Genome Medicine*, *11*(1), Article 70. https://doi.org/10.1186/s13073-019-0689-8

5. Dominguez-Valentin, M., Sampson, J. R., Seppälä, T. T., ten Broeke, S. W., Plazzer, J. P., Nakken, S., ... & Møller, P. (2019). Survival by colon cancer stage and screening

interval in Lynch syndrome: A prospective Lynch syndrome database report. *Hereditary Cancer in Clinical Practice, 17*, Article 28. https://doi.org/10.1186/s13053-019-0127-3

6. Eraslan, G., Avsec, Ž., Gagneur, J., & Theis, F. J. (2019). Deep learning: New computational modelling techniques for genomics. *Nature Reviews Genetics, 20*(7), 389–403. https://doi.org/10.1038/s41576-019-0122-6
7. Green, E. D., Gunter, C., Biesecker, L. G., Di Francesco, V., Easter, C. L., Feingold, E. A., Felsenfeld, A. L., Kaufman, D. J., Ostrander, E. A., Pavan, W. J., Phillippy, A. M., Wise, A. L., Dayal, J. G., Kish, B. J., Mandich, A., Wellington, C. R., Wetterstrand, K. A., Buccini, S. A., Garvey, L. D., ... Manolio, T. A. (2020). Strategic vision for improving human health at The Forefront of Genomics. *Nature, 586*(7831), 683–692. https://doi.org/10.1038/s41586-020-2817-4
8. Ho, D., Quake, S. R., McCabe, E. R. B., Chng, W. J., Chow, E. K., Ding, X., Gelb, B. D., Ginsburg, G. S., Hassenstab, J., Ho, C. M., Mobley, W. C., Nolan, G. P., Rosen, S. T., Tan, P., Yen, Y., & Zarrinpar, A. (2020). Enabling technologies for personalized and precision medicine. *Trends in Biotechnology, 38*(5), 497–518. https://doi.org/10.1016/j.tibtech.2019.12.021
9. Johnson, K. B., Wei, W. Q., Weeraratne, D., Frisse, M. E., Misulis, K., Rhee, K., Zhao, J., & Snowdon, J. L. (2021). Precision medicine, AI, and the future of personalized health care. *Clinical and Translational Science, 14*(1), 86–93. https://doi.org/10.1111/cts.12884

10. Klein, M. E., Parvez, M. M., & Shin, J. G. (2017). Clinical implementation of pharmacogenomics for personalized precision medicine: Barriers and solutions. *Journal of Pharmaceutical Sciences, 106*(9), 2368–2379. https://doi.org/10.1016/j.xphs.2017.04.051

11. Lauschke, V. M., Milani, L., & Ingelman-Sundberg, M. (2018). Pharmacogenomic biomarkers for improved drug therapy—Recent progress and future developments. *The AAPS Journal, 20*, Article 4. https://doi.org/10.1208/s12248-017-0161-x

12. Livingston, G., Huntley, J., Liu, K. Y., Costafreda, S. G., Selbæk, G., Alladi, S., Ames, D., Banerjee, S., Burns, A., Brayne, C., Fox, N. C., Ferri, C. P., Gitlin, L. N., Howard, R., Kales, H. C., Kivimäki, M., Larson, E. B., Nakasujja, N., Rockwood, K., ... Mukadam, N. (2024). Dementia prevention, intervention, and care: 2024 report of the Lancet standing Commission. *The Lancet, 404*(10452), 572–628. https://doi.org/10.1016/S0140-6736(24)01296-0

13. National Comprehensive Cancer Network. (2023). *NCCN clinical practice guidelines in oncology: Genetic/familial high-risk assessment: Breast, ovarian, and pancreatic* (Version 2.2024). https://www.nccn.org/guidelines/guidelines-detail?category=2&id=1503

14. National Human Genome Research Institute. (2023). *The cost of sequencing a human genome.* https://www.genome.gov/about-genomics/fact-sheets/Sequencing-Human-Genome-cost

15. Norwitz, N. G., Saif, N., Ariza, I. E., & Isaacson, R. S. (2021). Precision nutrition for Alzheimer's prevention in

ApoE4 carriers. *Nutrients, 13*(4), Article 1362. https://doi.org/10.3390/nu13041362

16. Relling, M. V., & Evans, W. E. (2015). Pharmacogenomics in the clinic. *Nature, 526*(7573), 343–350. https://doi.org/10.1038/nature15817
17. Shendure, J., Findlay, G. M., & Snyder, M. W. (2019). Genomic medicine–Progress, pitfalls, and promise. *Cell, 177*(1), 45–57. https://doi.org/10.1016/j.cell.2019.02.003
18. Sherzai, D., & Sherzai, A. (2017). *The Alzheimer's solution: A breakthrough program to prevent and reverse the symptoms of cognitive decline at every age.* HarperOne.
19. Stark, Z., Dolman, L., Manolio, T. A., Ozenberger, B., Hill, S. L., Caulfied, M. J., Levy, Y., Glazer, D., Wilson, J., Lawler, M., Boughtwood, T., Braithwaite, J., Goodhand, P., Birney, E., & North, K. N. (2019). Integrating genomics into healthcare: A global responsibility. *American Journal of Human Genetics, 104*(1), 13–20. https://doi.org/10.1016/j.ajhg.2018.11.014
20. Topol, E. J. (2019). High-performance medicine: The convergence of human and artificial intelligence. *Nature Medicine, 25*(1), 44–56. https://doi.org/10.1038/s41591-018-0300-7
21. U.S. Food and Drug Administration. (2023). *Table of pharmacogenetic associations.* https://www.fda.gov/medical-devices/precision-medicine/table-pharmacogenetic-associations
22. Zanger, U. M., & Schwab, M. (2013). Cytochrome P450 enzymes in drug metabolism: Regulation of gene

expression, enzyme activities, and impact of genetic variation. *Pharmacology & Therapeutics, 138*(1), 103–141. https://doi.org/10.1016/j.pharmthera.2012.12.007

23. Zou, J., Huss, M., Abid, A., Mohammadi, P., Torkamani, A., & Telenti, A. (2019). A primer on deep learning in genomics. *Nature Genetics, 51*(1), 12–18. https://doi.org/10.1038/s41588-018-0295-5

## Part 2: Smart Health Solutions

### Heart Health and AI: Partners in Prevention

1. American Heart Association. (2020). Heart disease and stroke statistics—2020 update: A report from the American Heart Association. *Circulation, 141*(9), e139–e596. https://doi.org/10.1161/CIR.0000000000000757
2. Attia, Z. I., Noseworthy, P. A., Lopez-Jimenez, F., Asirvatham, S. J., Deshmukh, A. J., Gersh, B. J., Carter, R. E., Yao, X., Rabinstein, A. A., Erickson, B. J., Kapa, S., & Friedman, P. A. (2019). An artificial intelligence-enabled ECG algorithm for the identification of patients with atrial fibrillation during sinus rhythm: A retrospective analysis of outcome prediction. *The Lancet, 394*(10201), 861–867. https://doi.org/10.1016/S0140-6736(19)31721-0
3. DiNicolantonio, J. J., & O'Keefe, J. H. (2017). Added sugars drive coronary heart disease via insulin resistance and hyperinsulinaemia: A new paradigm. *Open Heart, 4*(2), Article e000729. https://doi.org/10.1136/openhrt-2017-000729
4. Ference, B. A., Ginsberg, H. N., Graham, I., Ray, K. K., Packard, C. J., Bruckert, E., Hegele, R. A., Krauss,

R. M., Raal, F. J., Schunkert, H., Watts, G. F., Borén, J., Fazio, S., Horton, J. D., Masana, L., Nicholls, S. J., Nordestgaard, B. G., van de Sluis, B., Taskinen, M.-R., ... Catapano, A. L. (2017). Low-density lipoproteins cause atherosclerotic cardiovascular disease: Pathophysiological, genetic, and therapeutic insights: A consensus statement from the European Atherosclerosis Society Consensus Panel. *European Heart Journal, 38*(32), 2459–2472. https://doi.org/10.1093/eurheartj/ehx144

5. Grandner, M. A., Jackson, N., Gerstner, J. R., & Knutson, K. L. (2013). Dietary nutrients associated with short and long sleep duration: Data from a nationally representative sample. *Appetite, 64*, 71–80. https://doi.org/10.1016/j.appet.2013.01.004
6. Greer, S. M., Goldstein, A. N., & Walker, M. P. (2013). The impact of sleep deprivation on food desire in the human brain. *Nature Communications, 4*, Article 2259. https://doi.org/10.1038/ncomms3259
7. Hu, F. B., & Malik, V. S. (2010). Sugar-sweetened beverages and risk of obesity and type 2 diabetes: Epidemiologic evidence. *Physiology & Behavior, 100*(1), 47–54. https://doi.org/10.1016/j.physbeh.2010.01.036
8. Javaheri, S., & Redline, S. (2017). Insomnia and risk of cardiovascular disease. *Chest, 152*(2), 435–444. https://doi.org/10.1016/j.chest.2017.01.026
9. Khera, A. V., Chaffin, M., Aragam, K. G., Haas, M. E., Roselli, C., Choi, S. H., Natarajan, P., Lander, E. S., Lubitz, S. A., Ellinor, P. T., & Kathiresan, S. (2018). Genome-wide polygenic scores for common diseases

identify individuals with risk equivalent to monogenic mutations. *Nature Genetics, 50*(9), 1219–1224. https://doi.org/10.1038/s41588-018-0183-z

10. Lear, S. A., Hu, W., Rangarajan, S., Gasevic, D., Leong, D., Iqbal, R., Casanova, A., Swaminathan, S., Anjana, R. M., Kumar, R., Rosengren, A., Wei, L., Yang, W., Chuangshi, W., Huaxing, L., ... Yusuf, S. (2017). The effect of physical activity on mortality and cardiovascular disease in 130,000 people from 17 high-income, middle-income, and low-income countries: The PURE study. *The Lancet, 390*(10113), 2643–2654. https://doi.org/10.1016/S0140-6736(17)31634-3
11. Leng, W. D., Zeng, X. T., Kwong, J. S., & Hua, X. P. (2015). Periodontal disease and risk of coronary heart disease: An updated meta-analysis of prospective cohort studies. *International Journal of Cardiology, 201*, 469–472. https://doi.org/10.1016/j.ijcard.2015.07.087
12. Libby, P., Buring, J. E., Badimon, L., Hansson, G. K., Deanfield, J., Bittencourt, M. S., Tokgözoğlu, L., & Lewis, E. F. (2019). Atherosclerosis. *Nature Reviews: Disease Primers, 5*(1), Article 56. https://doi.org/10.1038/s41572-019-0106-z
13. Libby, P., Ridker, P. M., & Maseri, A. (2002). Inflammation and atherosclerosis. *Circulation, 105*(9), 1135–1143. https://doi.org/10.1161/hc0902.104353
14. Libby, P., Ridker, P. M., Hansson, G. K., & Atherothrombosis, L. T. N. (2009). Inflammation in atherosclerosis: From pathophysiology to practice. *Journal of the American College of Cardiology, 54*(23), 2129–2138. https://doi.org/10.1016/j.jacc.2009.09.009

15. Makarem, N., Zuraikat, F. M., Redline, S., Aggarwal, B., Jelic, S., & St-Onge, M. P. (2022). Redefining cardiovascular health to include sleep: Prospective associations with cardiovascular disease in the MESA Sleep Study. *Journal of the American Heart Association, 11*(9), Article e025252. https://doi.org/10.1161/JAHA.122.025252

16. Ridker, P. M., Everett, B. M., Thuren, T., MacFadyen, J. G., Chang, W. H., Ballantyne, C., Fonseca, F., Nicolau, J., Koenig, W., Anker, S. D., Kastelein, J. J. P., Cornel, J. H., Pais, P., Pella, D., Genest, J., ... Glynn, R. J. (2017). Anti-inflammatory therapy with canakinumab for atherosclerotic disease. *New England Journal of Medicine, 377*(12), 1119–1131. https://doi.org/10.1056/NEJMoa1707914

17. St-Onge, M.-P., Grandner, M. A., Brown, D., Conroy, M. B., Jean-Louis, G., Coons, M., & Bhatt, D. L. (2016). Sleep duration and quality: Impact on lifestyle behaviors and cardiometabolic health: A scientific statement from the American Heart Association. *Circulation, 134*(18), e367–e386. https://doi.org/10.1161/CIR.0000000000000444

18. Tison, G. H., Sanchez, J. M., Ballinger, B., Singh, A., Olgin, J. E., Pletcher, M. J., Vittinghoff, E., Lee, E. S., Fan, S. M., Gladstone, R. A., Mikell, C., Sohoni, N., Hsieh, J., & Marcus, G. M. (2018). Passive detection of atrial fibrillation using a commercially available smartwatch. *JAMA Cardiology, 3*(5), 409–416. https://doi.org/10.1001/jamacardio.2018.0136

19. Virani, S. S., Alonso, A., Benjamin, E. J., Bittencourt, M. S., Callaway, C. W., Carson, A. P., Chamberlain, A.

M., Chang, A. R., Cheng, S., Delling, F. N., Djousse, L., Elkind, M. S. V., Ferguson, J. F., Fornage, M., Khan, S. S., ... Tsao, C. W. (2021). Heart disease and stroke statistics—2021 update: A report from the American Heart Association. *Circulation, 143*(8), e254–e743. https://doi.org/10.1161/CIR.0000000000000950

20. World Health Organization. (2024). *Cardiovascular diseases* [Fact sheet]. https://www.who.int/news-room/fact-sheets/detail/cardiovascular-diseases-(cvds)

21. Yang, Q., Zhang, Z., Gregg, E. W., Flanders, W. D., Merritt, R., & Hu, F. B. (2014). Added sugar intake and cardiovascular diseases mortality among US adults. *JAMA Internal Medicine, 174*(4), 516–524. https://doi.org/10.1001/jamainternmed.2013.13563

### The Role of AI in the Quiet Struggle of Mental Health

1. Abd-Alrazaq, A. A., Alajlani, M., Alalwan, A. A., Bewick, B. M., Gardner, P., & Househ, M. (2019). An overview of the features of chatbots in mental health: A scoping review. *International Journal of Medical Informatics, 132*, Article 103978. https://doi.org/10.1016/j.ijmedinf.2019.103978

2. Abd-Alrazaq, A. A., Rababeh, A., Alajlani, M., Bewick, B. M., & Househ, M. (2020). Effectiveness and safety of using chatbots to improve mental health: Systematic review and meta-analysis. *Journal of Medical Internet Research, 22*(7), Article e16021. https://doi.org/10.2196/16021

3. Babor, T. F., Higgins-Biddle, J. C., Saunders, J. B., & Monteiro, M. G. (2001). *AUDIT: The Alcohol Use*

*Disorders Identification Test*. World Health Organization. https://www.who.int/publications/i/item/audit-the-alcohol-use-disorders-identification-test-guidelines-for-use-in-primary-health-care

4. Baumeister, R. F., & Tierney, J. (2011). *Willpower: Rediscovering the greatest human strength*. Penguin Press.

5. Bovin, M. J., Marx, B. P., Weathers, F. W., Gallagher, M. W., Rodriguez, P., Schnurr, P. P., & Keane, T. M. (2016). Psychometric properties of the PTSD Checklist for DSM-5 (PCL-5). *Psychological Assessment, 28*(11), 1379–1391. https://doi.org/10.1037/pas0000254

6. Demyttenaere, K., Bruffaerts, R., Posada-Villa, J., Gasquet, I., Kovess, V., Lepine, J. P., Angermeyer, M. C., Bernert, S., de Girolamo, G., Morosini, P., Polidori, G., Kikkawa, T., Kawakami, N., Ono, Y., Takeshima, T., Uda, H., Karam, E. G., Fayyad, J. A., Karam, A. N., & WHO World Mental Health Survey Consortium. (2004). Prevalence, severity, and unmet need for treatment of mental disorders in the World Health Organization World Mental Health Surveys. *JAMA, 291*(21), 2581–2590. https://doi.org/10.1001/jama.291.21.2581

7. Drevets, W. C., Price, J. L., & Furey, M. L. (2008). Brain structural and functional abnormalities in mood disorders: Implications for neurocircuitry models of depression. *Brain Structure and Function, 213*(1–2), 93–118. https://doi.org/10.1007/s00429-008-0189-x

8. Edelson, J., & Tech Justice Law Project. (2025, August 26). *Complaint for damages and injunctive relief* [Legal filing]. Superior Court of California, County of San Francisco.

9. Fitzpatrick, K. K., Darcy, A., & Vierhile, M. (2017). Delivering cognitive behavior therapy to young adults with symptoms of depression and anxiety using a fully automated conversational agent (Woebot): A randomized controlled trial. *JMIR Mental Health, 4*(2), Article e19. https://doi.org/10.2196/mental.7785

10. Harvard Medical School. (2023). Half of world's population will experience a mental health disorder. https://hms.harvard.edu/news/half-worlds-population-will-experience-mental-health-disorder

11. Hirschfeld, R. M. A., Williams, J. B. W., Spitzer, R. L., Calabrese, J. R., Flynn, L., Keck, P. E., Jr., Lewis, L., McElroy, S. L., Post, R. M., Rapport, D. J., Russell, J. M., Sachs, G. S., & Zajecka, J. (2000). Development and validation of a screening instrument for bipolar spectrum disorder: The Mood Disorder Questionnaire. *American Journal of Psychiatry, 157*(11), 1873–1875. https://doi.org/10.1176/appi.ajp.157.11.1873

12. Ilardi, S. S. (2009). *The depression cure: The 6-step program to beat depression without drugs*. Da Capo Press.

13. Inzlicht, M., & Schmeichel, B. J. (2012). What is ego depletion? Toward a mechanistic revision of the resource model of self-control. *Perspectives on Psychological Science, 7*(5), 450–463. https://doi.org/10.1177/1745691612454134

14. Kroenke, K., Spitzer, R. L., & Williams, J. B. W. (2001). The PHQ-9: Validity of a brief depression severity measure. *Journal of General Internal Medicine, 16*(9), 606–613. https://doi.org/10.1046/j.1525-1497.2001.016009606.x

15. Mohr, D. C., Zhang, M., & Schueller, S. M. (2017). Personal sensing: Understanding mental health using ubiquitous sensors and machine learning. *Annual Review of Clinical Psychology, 13,* 23–47. https://doi.org/10.1146/annurev-clinpsy-032816-044949

16. NBC News. (2025, August 26). *The family of teenager who died by suicide alleges OpenAI's ChatGPT is to blame.* https://www.nbcnews.com/tech/tech-news/family-teenager-died-suicide-alleges-openais-chatgpt-blame-rcna226147

17. OpenAI. (2025, August 26). *Helping people when they need it most* [Blog post]. https://openai.com/blog/helping-people-when-they-need-it-most

18. Spitzer, R. L., Kroenke, K., Williams, J. B. W., & Löwe, B. (2006). A brief measure for assessing generalized anxiety disorder: The GAD-7. *Archives of Internal Medicine, 166*(10), 1092–1097. https://doi.org/10.1001/archinte.166.10.1092

19. Sullivan, P. F., Neale, M. C., & Kendler, K. S. (2000). Genetic epidemiology of major depression: Review and meta-analysis. *American Journal of Psychiatry, 157*(10), 1552–1562. https://doi.org/10.1176/appi.ajp.157.10.1552

20. Walker, M. P., & van der Helm, E. (2009). Overnight therapy? The role of sleep in emotional brain processing. *Psychological Bulletin, 135*(5), 731–748. https://doi.org/10.1037/a0016570

## Using AI to Address Obesity

1. American Cancer Society. (2025). *Cancer facts & figures 2025.* https://www.cancer.org/research/

cancer-facts-statistics/all-cancer-facts-figures/2025-cancer-facts-figures.html

2. Aroda, V. R., Edelstein, S. L., Goldberg, R. B., Knowler, W. C., Marcovina, S. M., Orchard, T. J., Bray, G. A., Schade, D. S., Temprosa, M. G., White, N. H., Crandall, J. P., & Diabetes Prevention Program Research Group. (2016). Long-term metformin use and vitamin B12 deficiency in the Diabetes Prevention Program Outcomes Study. *The Journal of Clinical Endocrinology & Metabolism, 101*(4), 1754–1761. https://doi.org/10.1210/jc.2015-3754
3. Aronne, L. J., Wadden, T. A., Peterson, C., Winslow, D., Odeh, S., & Gadde, K. M. (2013). Evaluation of phentermine and topiramate versus phentermine/topiramate extended-release in obese adults. *Obesity, 21*(11), 2163–2171. https://doi.org/10.1002/oby.20584
4. Bray, G. A., Heisel, W. E., Afshin, A., Jensen, M. D., Dietz, W. H., Long, M., Kushner, R. F., Daniels, S. R., Wadden, T. A., Tsai, A. G., Hu, F. B., Jakicic, J. M., Ryan, D. H., Wolfe B. M., & Inge, T. H. (2018). The science of obesity management: An Endocrine Society scientific statement. *Endocrine Reviews, 39*(2), 79–132. https://doi.org/10.1210/er.2017-00253
5. Campbell, J. E., & Drucker, D. J. (2013). Pharmacology, physiology, and mechanisms of incretin hormone action. *Cell Metabolism, 17*(6), 819–837. https://doi.org/10.1016/j.cmet.2013.04.008
6. Centers for Disease Control and Prevention. (2023). *Adult obesity facts.* https://www.cdc.gov/obesity/adult-obesity-facts/index.html

7. Centers for Disease Control and Prevention. (2024, May 15). *National diabetes statistics report*. U.S. Department of Health and Human Services. https://www.cdc.gov/diabetes/php/data-research/index.html

8. Chao, A. M., Quigley, K. M., & Wadden, T. A. (2021). Dietary interventions for obesity: Clinical and mechanistic findings. *Journal of Clinical Investigation, 131*(1), Article e140065. https://doi.org/10.1172/JCI140065

9. Clear, J. (2018). *Atomic habits: An easy & proven way to build good habits & break bad ones*. Avery.

10. Fadhil, A., Wang, Y., & Reiterer, H. (2019). Assistive conversational agent for health coaching: A validation study. *Methods of Information in Medicine, 58*(1), 9–23. https://doi.org/10.1055/s-0039-1688757

11. Fogg, B. J. (2019). *Tiny habits: The small changes that change everything*. Houghton Mifflin Harcourt.

12. Hari, J. (2024). *Magic pill: The extraordinary benefits and disturbing risks of the new weight-loss drugs*. Crown.

13. Jospe, M. R., Roy, M., Brown, R. C., Haszard, J. J., Meredith-Jones, K., Fangupo, L. J., Osborne, H., Fleming, E. A., & Taylor, R. W. (2020). Intermittent fasting, Paleolithic, or Mediterranean diets in the real world: Exploratory secondary analyses of a weight-loss trial that included choice of diet and exercise. *The American Journal of Clinical Nutrition, 111*(3), 503–514. https://doi.org/10.1093/ajcn/nqz330

14. Kahan, S., & Manson, J. E. (2019). Obesity treatment, beyond the guidelines: Practical suggestions for

clinical practice. *JAMA, 321*(14), 1349–1350. https://doi.org/10.1001/jama.2019.2352

15. Kramer, C. K., Zinman, B., & Retnakaran, R. (2013). Are metabolically healthy overweight and obesity benign conditions? A systematic review and meta-analysis. *Annals of Internal Medicine, 159*(11), 758–769. https://doi.org/10.7326/0003-4819-159-11-201312030-00008

16. Lentferink, A. J., Oldenhuis, H. K., de Groot, M., Polstra, L., Velthuijsen, H., & van Gemert-Pijnen, J. E. (2017). Key components in eHealth interventions combining self-tracking and persuasive eCoaching to promote a healthier lifestyle: A scoping review. *Journal of Medical Internet Research, 19*(8), Article e277. https://doi.org/10.2196/jmir.7288

17. Lorenz, K. A., Yeshurun, S., Aziz, R., Ortiz-Delatorre, J., Bagley, J. R., Mor, M., & Kern, M. (2021). A handheld metabolic device (Lumen) to measure fuel utilization in healthy young adults: Device validation study. *Interactive Journal of Medical Research, 10*(2), Article e25371. https://doi.org/10.2196/25371

18. Ludwig, D. S., & Ebbeling, C. B. (2018). The carbohydrate-insulin model of obesity: Beyond "calories in, calories out". *JAMA Internal Medicine, 178*(8), 1098–1103. https://doi.org/10.1001/jamainternmed.2018.2933

19. Mason, S. M., Flint, A. J., Roberts, A. L., Agnew-Blais, J., Koenen, K. C., & Rich-Edwards, J. W. (2014). Posttraumatic stress disorder symptoms and food addiction in women by timing and type of trauma exposure. *JAMA Psychiatry, 71*(11), 1271–1278. https://doi.org/10.1001/jamapsychiatry.2014.1208

20. Molina-Montes, E., Salamanca-Fernández, E., Garcia-Villanova, B., & Sánchez, M. J. (2020). The impact of plant-based dietary patterns on cancer-related outcomes: A rapid review and meta-analysis. *Nutrients, 12*(7), Article 2010. https://doi.org/10.3390/nu12072010

21. Moss, M. (2013). *Salt sugar fat: How the food giants hooked us*. Random House.

22. National Institute of Diabetes and Digestive and Kidney Diseases. (2025). *Insulin resistance & prediabetes*. U.S. Department of Health and Human Services, National Institutes of Health. https://www.niddk.nih.gov/health-information/diabetes/overview/what-is-diabetes/prediabetes-insulin-resistance

23. PBS NewsHour. (2023, May 23). *Black people are more likely to develop Alzheimer's than white people, CDC says.* https://www.pbs.org/newshour/health/black-people-are-more-likely-to-develop-alzheimers-than-white-people-cdc-says

24. Sattar, N., Preiss, D., Murray, H. M., Welsh, P., Buckley, B. M., de Craen, A. J., Seshasai, S. R., McMurray, J. J., Freeman, D. J., Jukema, J. W., Macfarlane, P. W., Packard, C. J., Stott, D. J., Westendorp, R. G., Shepherd, J., Davis, B. R., Pressel, S. L., Marchioli, R., Marfisi, R. M., ... Ford, I. (2010). Statins and risk of incident diabetes: A collaborative meta-analysis of randomised statin trials. *Lancet (London, England), 375*(9716), 735–742. https://doi.org/10.1016/S0140-6736(09)61965-6

25. Seidelmann, S. B., Claggett, B., Cheng, S., Henglin, M., Shah, A., Steffen, L. M., Folsom, A. R., Rimm, E.

B., Willett, W. C., & Solomon, S. D. (2018). Dietary carbohydrate intake and mortality: A prospective cohort study and meta-analysis. *The Lancet Public Health, 3*(9), e419–e428. https://doi.org/10.1016/S2468-2667(18)30135-X

26. Shapira, S. N., & Seale, P. (2019). Transcriptional control of brown and beige fat development and function. *Obesity (Silver Spring, Md.), 27*(1), 13–21. https://doi.org/10.1002/oby.22334

27. Spiegel, K., Tasali, E., Leproult, R., & Van Cauter, E. (2009). Effects of poor and short sleep on glucose metabolism and obesity risk. *Nature Reviews Endocrinology, 5*(5), 253–261. https://doi.org/10.1038/nrendo.2009.23

28. Tong, H. L., Coiera, E., & Laranjo, L. (2018). Using a mobile social networking app to promote physical activity: A qualitative study of users' perspectives. *Journal of Medical Internet Research, 20*(12), Article e11439. https://doi.org/10.2196/11439

29. Trexler, E. T., Smith-Ryan, A. E., & Norton, L. E. (2014). Metabolic adaptation to weight loss: implications for the athlete. *Journal of the International Society of Sports Nutrition, 11*, Article 7. https://doi.org/10.1186/1550-2783-11-7

30. Trouwborst, I., Costabile, G., Esser, D., Blaak, E. E., Saris, W. H. M., Munsters, M. J. M., Virgili, F., Tuohy, K., Delafiore, G., Bozzetto, L., Giacco, R., Rivellese, A. A., Riccardi, G., Mensink, R. P., & Afman, L. A. (2023). Cardiometabolic health improvements upon dietary intervention are driven by tissue-specific insulin resistance phenotype: A precision nutrition trial. *Cell*

*Metabolism, 35*(1), 71–83.e5. https://doi.org/10.1016/j.cmet.2022.12.002

31. UK Prospective Diabetes Study Group. (1998). Effect of intensive blood-glucose control with metformin on complications in overweight patients with type 2 diabetes (UKPDS 34). *The Lancet, 352*(9131), 854–865. https://doi.org/10.1016/S0140-6736(98)07037-8

32. Wadden, T. A., Tronieri, J. S., & Butryn, M. L. (2020). Lifestyle modification approaches for the treatment of obesity in adults. *American Psychologist, 75*(2), 235–251. https://doi.org/10.1037/amp0000517

33. Wilding, J. P. H., Batterham, R. L., Calanna, S., Davies, M., Van Gaal, L. F., Lingvay, I., McGowan, B. M., Rosenstock, J., Tran, M. T. D., Wadden, T. A., Wharton, S., Yokote, K., Zeuthen, N., & Kushner, R. F. (2021). Once-weekly semaglutide in adults with overweight or obesity. *New England Journal of Medicine, 384*(11), 989–1002. https://doi.org/10.1056/NEJMoa2032183

34. Wing, R. R., & Phelan, S. (2005). Long-term weight loss maintenance. The *American Journal of Clinical Nutrition, 82*(1), 222S–225S. https://doi.org/10.1093/ajcn/82.1.222S

35. World Health Organization Expert Consultation. (2004). Appropriate body-mass index for Asian populations and its implications for policy and intervention strategies. *The Lancet, 363*(9403), 157–163. https://doi.org/10.1016/S0140-6736(03)15268-3

36. World Health Organization. (2019, April 21). *Classification of diabetes mellitus* [Brochure].

https://www.who.int/publications/i/item/classification-of-diabetes-mellitus

37. World Health Organization. (2023). *Obesity and overweight.* https://www.who.int/news-room/fact-sheets/detail/obesity-and-overweight

38. Yanovski, S. Z., & Yanovski, J. A. (2018). Toward precision approaches for the prevention and treatment of obesity. *JAMA, 319*(3), 223–224. https://doi.org/10.1001/jama.2017.20051

39. Yeary, K. H. K., Cornell, C. E., Moore, P. C., Gauss, C. H., Prewitt, T. E., & Turner, J. (2020). The WORD: Outcomes of a behavioral weight loss maintenance effectiveness trial in rural Black adults of faith. *Obesity, 28*(3), 510–520. https://doi.org/10.1002/oby.22717

40. Zeevi, D., Korem, T., Zmora, N., Israeli, D., Rothschild, D., Weinberger, A., Ben-Yacov, O., Lador, D., Avnit-Sagi, T., Lotan-Pompan, M., Suez, J., Mahdi, J. A., Matot, E., Malka, G., Kosower, N., Rein, M., Zilberman-Schapira, G., Dohnalová, L., Pevsner-Fischer, M., ... Segal, E. (2015). Personalized nutrition by prediction of glycemic responses. *Cell, 163*(5), 1079–1094. https://doi.org/10.1016/j.cell.2015.11.001

### Dementia and AI: Prevention, Detection, and Management

1. Alzheimer's Association. (2023). *2023 Alzheimer's disease facts and figures.* https://www.alz.org/alzheimers-dementia/facts-figures

2. Alzheimer's disease facts and figures. (2023) *Alzheimer's & Dementia, 19*(4), 1598–1695. https://doi.org/10.1002/alz.13016

3. Barnes, L. L., & Bennett, D. A. (2014). Alzheimer's disease in African Americans: Risk factors and challenges for the future. *Health Affairs, 33*(4), 580–586. https://doi.org/10.1377/hlthaff.2013.1353

4. Brandt, J., Buchholz, A., Henry-Barron, B., Vizthum, D., Avramopoulos, D., & Cervenka, M. C. (2019). Preliminary report on the feasibility and efficacy of the modified Atkins diet for treatment of mild cognitive impairment and early Alzheimer's disease. *Journal of Alzheimer's Disease, 68*(3), 969–981. https://doi.org/10.3233/JAD-180995 (Available at: https://pubmed.ncbi.nlm.nih.gov/30856112/)

5. Buchholz, A., Deme, P., Betz, J. F., Brandt, J., Haughey, N., & Cervenka, M. C. (2024). A randomized feasibility trial of the modified Atkins diet in older adults with mild cognitive impairment due to Alzheimer's disease. *Frontiers in Endocrinology, 15*, Article 1182519. https://doi.org/10.3389/fendo.2024.1182519

6. Centers for Disease Control and Prevention. (2024a). *Alzheimer's disease and healthy aging data portal.* https://www.cdc.gov/healthy-aging-data/index.html

7. Centers for Disease Control and Prevention. (2024b). *National diabetes statistics report.* U.S. Department of Health and Human Services. https://www.cdc.gov/diabetes/php/data-research/index.html

8. Demetriou, A., Makris, N., & Spanoudis, G. (2018). In defense of a developmental theory of intelligence: Response to the commentators. *Human Development, 61*(2), 138–143. https://doi.org/10.1159/000489840

9. Eyigoz, E., Mathur, S., Santamaria, M., Cecchi, G., & Naylor, M. (2020). Linguistic markers predict onset of Alzheimer's disease. *eClinicalMedicine*, *28*, Article 100583. https://doi.org/10.1016/j.eclinm.2020.100583

10. Huang, L. C., Lee, M. Y., Chien, C. F., Chang, Y. P., Li, K. Y., & Yang, Y. H. (2023). Age and sex differences in the association between APOE genotype and Alzheimer's disease in a Taiwan Chinese population. *Frontiers in Aging Neuroscience*, *15*, Article 1246592. https://doi.org/10.3389/fnagi.2023.1246592

11. Husain, M., Zetterberg, H., & Schott, J. M. (2022). Blood biomarkers for Alzheimer's disease: Towards clinical implementation. *The Lancet Neurology*, *21*(1), 66–77. https://doi.org/10.1016/S1474-4422(21)00361-6

12. Kourtis, L. C., Regele, O. B., Wright, J. M., & Jones, G. B. (2019). Digital biomarkers for Alzheimer's disease: The mobile/wearable devices opportunity. *NPJ Digital Medicine*, *2*, Article 9. https://doi.org/10.1038/s41746-019-0084-2

13. Langa, K. M., & Levine, D. A. (2014). The diagnosis and management of mild cognitive impairment: A clinical review. *JAMA*, *312*(23), 2551–2561. https://doi.org/10.1001/jama.2014.13806

14. Livingston, G., Huntley, J., Sommerlad, A., Ames, D., Ballard, C., Banerjee, S., Brayne, C., Burns, A., Cohen-Mansfield, J., Cooper, C., Costafreda, S. G., Dias, A., Fox, N., Gitlin, L. N., Howard, R., Kales, H. C., Kivimäki, M., Larson, E. B., Ogunniyi, A., ... Mukadam, N. (2020). Dementia prevention, intervention, and care: 2020 report of the Lancet Commission. *The*

*Lancet*, *396*(10248), 413–446. https://doi.org/10.1016/S0140-6736(20)30367-6

15. Marciniak, R., Sheardova, K., Čermáková, P., Hudeček, D., Šumec, R., & Hort, J. (2022). Effect of meditation on cognitive functions in context of aging and neurodegenerative diseases. *Frontiers in Behavioral Neuroscience*, *8*, Article 17. https://doi.org/10.3389/fnbeh.2014.00017

16. Morris, M. C., Tangney, C. C., Wang, Y., Sacks, F. M., Barnes, L. L., Bennett, D. A., & Aggarwal, N. T. (2015). MIND diet slows cognitive decline with aging. *Alzheimer's & Dementia : The Journal of the Alzheimer's Association*, *11*(9), 1015–1022. https://doi.org/10.1016/j.jalz.2015.04.011

17. National Institute on Aging. (2023). *Preventing Alzheimer's disease: What do we know?* https://www.nia.nih.gov/health/alzheimers-and-dementia/preventing-alzheimers-disease-what-do-we-know

18. Patnode, C. D., Perdue, L. A., Rossom, R. C., Rushkin, M. C., Redmond, N., Thomas, R. G., & Lin, J. S. (2020). Screening for cognitive impairment in older adults: Updated evidence report and systematic review for the US Preventive Services Task Force. *JAMA*, *323*(8), 764–785. https://doi.org/10.1001/jama.2019.22258

19. PBS NewsHour. (2023, May 23). *Black people are more likely to develop Alzheimer's than white people, CDC says.* https://www.pbs.org/newshour/health/black-people-are-more-likely-to-develop-alzheimers-than-white-people-cdc-says

20. Piau, A., Wild, K., Mattek, N., & Kaye, J. (2019). Current state of digital biomarker technologies for real-life,

home-based monitoring of cognitive function for mild cognitive impairment to mild Alzheimer disease and implications for clinical care: Systematic review. *Journal of Medical Internet Research, 21*(8), Article e12785. https://doi.org/10.2196/12785

21. Sabbagh, M. N., Boada, M., Borson, S., Chilukuri, M., Doraiswamy, P. M., Dubois, B., Ingram, J., Iwata, A., Porsteinsson, A. P., Possin, K. L., Rabinovici, G. D., Vellas, B., Chao, S., Vergallo, A., & Hampel, H. (2020). Rationale for early diagnosis of mild cognitive impairment (MCI) supported by emerging digital technologies. *Journal of Prevention of Alzheimer's Disease, 7*(3), 158–164. https://doi.org/10.14283/jpad.2020.19

22. Sabbagh, M. N., Perez, A., Holland, T. M., Boustani, M., Peabody, S. R., Yaffe, K., et al. (2022). Primary prevention recommendations to reduce the risk of cognitive decline. *Alzheimer's & Dementia, 18*(8), 1569–1579. https://doi.org/10.1002/alz.12535

23. Scarmeas, N., Anastasiou, C. A., & Yannakoulia, M. (2018). Nutrition and prevention of cognitive impairment. *The Lancet Neurology, 17*(11), 1006–1015. https://doi.org/10.1016/S1474-4422(18)30338-7

24. Tsoi, K. K., Chan, J. Y., Hirai, H. W., Wong, S. Y., & Kwok, T. C. (2015). Cognitive tests to detect dementia: A systematic review and meta-analysis. *JAMA Internal Medicine, 175*(9), 1450–1458. https://doi.org/10.1001/jamainternmed.2015.2152

25. Vassilaki, M., Aakre, J. A., Mielke, M. M., Geda, Y. E., Kremers, W. K., Alhurani, R. E., Machulda, M. M., Knopman, D. S., Petersen, R. C., Lowe, V. J., Jack, C.

R., Jr., & Roberts, R. O. (2016). Multimorbidity and neuroimaging biomarkers among cognitively normal persons. *Neurology, 86*(22), 2077–2084. https://doi.org/10.1212/WNL.0000000000002624

26. Walker, M. (2017). *Why we sleep: Unlocking the power of sleep and dreams.* Scribner.
27. World Health Organization. (2019). *Adopting a healthy lifestyle helps reduce the risk of dementia.* https://www.who.int/news-room/detail/14-05-2019-adopting-a-healthy-lifestyle-helps-reduce-the-risk-of-dementia
28. Yaffe, K. (2019). Prevention of cognitive impairment with intensive systolic blood pressure control. *JAMA, 321*(6), 548–549. https://doi.org/10.1001/jama.2019.0008
29. Zhang, H., Greenwood, D. C., Risch, H. A., Bunce, D., Hardie, L. J., & Cade, J. E. (2021). Meat consumption and risk of incident dementia: Cohort study of 493,888 UK Biobank participants. *The American Journal of Clinical Nutrition, 114*(1), 175–184. https://doi.org/10.1093/ajcn/nqab028

## Breast Cancer and AI: How Technology Can Help Prevent and Treat

1. American Cancer Society. (2024). *Breast cancer facts & figures 2024-2025.* https://www.cancer.org/content/dam/cancer-org/research/cancer-facts-and-statistics/breast-cancer-facts-and-figures/2024/breast-cancer-facts-and-figures-2024.pdf
2. Boyd, N. F., Martin, L. J., Sun, L., Guo, H., Chiarelli, A., Hislop, G., Yaffe, M., & Minkin, S. (2006). Body size, mammographic density, and breast cancer risk. *Cancer*

*Epidemiology, Biomarkers & Prevention, 15*(11), 2086–2092. https://doi.org/10.1158/1055-9965.EPI-06-0345

3. Churpek, J. E., Walsh, T., Zheng, Y., Moton, Z., Thornton, A. M., Lee, M. K., Casadei, S., Watts, A., Neistadt, B., Churpek, M. M., Huo, D., Zvosec, C., Liu, F., Niu, Q., Marquez, R., Zhang, J., Fackenthal, J., King, M. C., & Olopade, O. I. (2015). Inherited predisposition to breast cancer among African American women. *Breast Cancer Research and Treatment, 149*(1), 31–39. https://doi.org/10.1007/s10549-014-3195-0
4. Ellsworth, D. L., Turner, C. E., & Ellsworth, R. E. (2019). A review of the hereditary component of triple negative breast cancer: High- and moderate-penetrance breast cancer genes, low-penetrance loci, and the role of nontraditional genetic elements. *Journal of Oncology, 2019*, Article 4382606. https://doi.org/10.1155/2019/4382606
5. Ferreira, P., Duarte, C., Almeida, A., Santos, M., Cardoso, M. J., & Cardoso, J. S. (2023). Artificial intelligence in breast cancer care—From diagnosis to follow-up: A systematic review. *Cancers, 15*(11), Article 2841. https://doi.org/10.3390/cancers15112841
6. Freeman, K., Geppert, J., Stinton, C., Todkill, D., Johnson, S., Clarke, A., & Taylor-Phillips, S. (2021). Use of artificial intelligence for image analysis in breast cancer screening programmes: Systematic review of test accuracy. *BMJ, 374*, Article n1872. https://doi.org/10.1136/bmj.n1872
7. Giaquinto, A. N., Sung, H., Miller, K. D., Kramer, J. L., Newman, L. A., Yang, L., Jemal, A., Lortet-Tieulent,

J., & Siegel, R. L. (2022). Breast cancer statistics, 2022. *CA: A Cancer Journal for Clinicians*, *72*(6), 524–541. https://doi.org/10.3322/caac.21754

8. Hernström, V., Josefsson, V., Sartor, H., Schmidt, D., Larsson, A.-M., Hofvind, S., Andersson, I., Rosso, A., Hagberg, O., & Lång, K. (2025). Screening performance and characteristics of breast cancer detected in the Mammography Screening with Artificial Intelligence trial (MASAI): A randomised, controlled, parallel-group, non-inferiority, single-blinded, screening accuracy study. *The Lancet Digital Health*, *7*(3), e175–e183. https://doi.org/10.1016/S2589-7500(24)00267-X
9. Hirko, K. A., Rocque, G., Reasor, E., Taye, A., Daly, A., Cutress, R. I., Copson, E. R., Lee, D.-W., Lee, K.-H., Im, S.-A., Park, Y. H., & Newman, L. A. (2022). The impact of race and ethnicity in breast cancer—disparities and implications for precision oncology. *BMC Medicine*, *20*(1), Article 72. https://doi.org/10.1186/s12916-022-02260-0
10. Hussain, S., Ali, M., Naseem, U., Nezhadmoghadam, F., Jatoi, M. A., Gulliver, T. A., & Tamez-Peña, J. G. (2024). Breast cancer risk prediction using machine learning: A systematic review. *Frontiers in Oncology*, *14*, Article 1343627. https://doi.org/10.3389/fonc.2024.1343627
11. Islami, F., Guerra, C. E., Minihan, A., Yabroff, K. R., Fedewa, S. A., Sloan, K., Wiedt, T. L., Thomson, B., Siegel, R. L., Nargis, N., Winn, R. A., Lacasse, L., Makaroff, L., Daniels, E. C., Patel, A. V., Cance, W. G., & Jemal, A. (2022). American Cancer Society's report on the status of cancer disparities in the United States, 2021. *CA: A*

*Cancer Journal for Clinicians*, *72*(2), 112–143. https://doi.org/10.3322/caac.21703

12. Jatoi, I., & Newman, L. A. (2022). The emergence of the racial disparity in U.S. breast-cancer mortality. *New England Journal of Medicine*, *386*(25), 2349–2352. https://doi.org/10.1056/NEJMp2200244

13. Kuchenbaecker, K. B., Hopper, J. L., Barnes, D. R., Phillips, K. A., Mooij, T. M., Roos-Blom, M. J., ... & Easton, D. F. (2017). Risks of breast, ovarian, and contralateral breast cancer for BRCA1 and BRCA2 mutation carriers. *JAMA*, *317*(23), 2402–2416. https://doi.org/10.1001/jama.2017.7112

14. Lee, J. H., Kim, K. H., Lee, E. H., Ahn, J. S., Ryu, J. K., Park, Y. M., Shin, G. W., Kim, Y. J., & Choi, H. Y. (2022). Improving the performance of radiologists using artificial intelligence-based detection support software for mammography: A multi-reader study. *Korean Journal of Radiology*, *23*(5), 505–516. https://doi.org/10.3348/kjr.2021.0476

15. Leibig, C., Brehmer, M., Bunk, S., Byng, D., Pinker, K., & Umutlu, L. (2022). Combining the strengths of radiologists and AI for breast cancer screening: A retrospective analysis. *The Lancet Digital Health*, *4*(7), e507–e519. https://doi.org/10.1016/S2589-7500(22)00070-X

16. McCormack, V. A., & dos Santos Silva, I. (2006). Breast density and parenchymal patterns as markers of breast cancer risk: A meta-analysis. *Cancer Epidemiology, Biomarkers & Prevention*, *15*(6), 1159–1169. https://doi.org/10.1158/1055-9965.EPI-06-0034

17. McKinney, S. M., Sieniek, M., Godbole, V., Godwin, J., Antropova, N., Ashrafian, H., Back, T., Chesus, M., Corrado, G. S., Darzi, A., Etemadi, M., Garcia-Vicente, F., Gilbert, F. J., Halling-Brown, M., Hassabis, D., Jansen, S., Karthikesalingam, A., Kelly, C. J., King, D., ... Shetty, S. (2020). International evaluation of an AI system for breast cancer screening. *Nature*, *577*(7788), 89–94. https://doi.org/10.1038/s41586-019-1799-6

18. Molina, Y., Kim, S., Berrios, N., & Calhoun, E. A. (2015). Medical mistrust and patient satisfaction with mammography: The mediating effects of perceived self-efficacy among navigated African American women. *Health Expectations*, *18*(6), 2941–2950. https://doi.org/10.1111/hex.12278

19. Monticciolo, D. L., Malak, S. F., Friedewald, S. M., Eby, P. R., Newell, M. S., Moy, L., Destounis, S., Leung, J. W. T., Hendrick, R. E., & Smetherman, D. (2021). Breast cancer screening recommendations inclusive of all women at average risk: Update from the ACR and Society of Breast Imaging. *Journal of the American College of Radiology*, *18*(9), 1280–1288. https://doi.org/10.1016/j.jacr.2021.04.021

20. National Cancer Institute. (2024). Cancer stat facts: Female breast cancer. Surveillance, Epidemiology, and End Results (SEER) Program. https://seer.cancer.gov/statfacts/html/breast.html

21. Newman, L. A., & Kaljee, L. M. (2017). Health disparities and triple-negative breast cancer in African American women: A review. *JAMA Surgery*, *152*(5), 485–493. https://doi.org/10.1001/jamasurg.2017.0005

22. Pal Choudhury, P., Wilcox, A. N., Brook, M. N., Zhang, Y., Ahearn, T., Orr, N., Coulson, P., Schoemaker, M. J., Jones, M. E., Gail, M. H., Swerdlow, A. J., Chatterjee, N., & Garcia-Closas, M. (2020). Comparative validation of breast cancer risk prediction models and projections for future risk stratification. *Journal of the National Cancer Institute, 112*(3), 278–285. https://doi.org/10.1093/jnci/djz113

23. Salim, M., Wåhlin, E., Dembrower, K., Azavedo, E., Foukakis, T., Liu, Y., Smith, K., Eklund, M., & Strand, F. (2020). External evaluation of 3 commercial artificial intelligence algorithms for independent assessment of screening mammograms. *JAMA Oncology, 6*(10), 1581–1588. https://doi.org/10.1001/jamaoncol.2020.3321

24. Siegel, R. L., Miller, K. D., Wagle, N. S., & Jemal, A. (2023). Cancer statistics, 2023. *CA: A Cancer Journal for Clinicians, 73*(1), 17–48. https://doi.org/10.3322/caac.21763

25. Silva, H. E. C., et al. (2023). The use of artificial intelligence tools in cancer detection compared to the traditional diagnostic imaging methods: An overview of the systematic reviews. *PLoS One, 18*(10), Article e0292063. https://doi.org/10.1371/journal.pone.0292063

26. Susan G. Komen. (2025). *Understanding breast cancer survival rates.* https://www.komen.org/breast-cancer/facts-statistics/breast-cancer-statistics/survival-rates/

27. U.S. Preventive Services Task Force, Owens, D. K., Davidson, K. W., Krist, A. H., Barry, M. J., Cabana, M., Caughey, A. B., Doubeni, C. A., Epling, J. W., Jr., Kubik,

M., Landefeld, C. S., Mangione, C. M., Pbert, L., Silverstein, M., Simon, M. A., Tseng, C. W., & Wong, J. B. (2019). Risk assessment, genetic counseling, and genetic testing for BRCA-related cancer: US Preventive Services Task Force recommendation statement. *JAMA, 322*(7), 652–665. https://doi.org/10.1001/jama.2019.10987

28. Wilkerson, A. D., Gentle, C. K., Ortega, C., & Al-Hilli, Z. (2024). Disparities in breast cancer care—How factors related to prevention, diagnosis, and treatment drive inequity. *Healthcare, 12*(4), Article 462. https://doi.org/10.3390/healthcare12040462

### Colon Cancer and AI: Your Partner for Prevention, Detection, and Treatment

1. Akimoto, N., Ugai, T., Zhong, R., Hamada, T., Fujiyoshi, K., Giannakis, M., Wu, K., Cao, Y., Ng, K., & Ogino, S. (2021). Rising incidence of early-onset colorectal cancer - a call to action. *Nature Reviews Clinical Oncology, 18*(4), 230–243. https://doi.org/10.1038/s41571-020-00445-1
2. American Cancer Society. (2023). *Colorectal cancer facts & figures 2023-2025*. https://www.cancer.org/content/dam/cancer-org/research/cancer-facts-and-statistics/colorectal-cancer-facts-and-figures/colorectal-cancer-facts-and-figures-2023.pdf
3. Augustus, G. J., & Ellis, N. A. (2018). Colorectal cancer disparity in African Americans: Risk factors and carcinogenic mechanisms. *American Journal of Pathology, 188*(2), 291–303. https://doi.org/10.1016/j.ajpath.2017.07.023

4. Carethers, J. M. (2021). Racial and ethnic disparities in colorectal cancer incidence and mortality. *Advances in Cancer Research, 151,* 197–229. https://doi.org/10.1016/bs.acr.2021.02.007

5. Changchien, E. M., Hawkins, M., Murday, M. E., & Griffin, J. A. (2014, August 21). *Is 10 years too long? Development of interval colorectal cancer despite following recommended colonoscopic guidelines.* SAGES. https://www.sages.org/meetings/annual-meeting/abstracts-archive/is-10-years-too-long-development-of-interval-colorectal-cancer-despite-following-recommended-colonoscopic-guidelines/

6. Cornish, A. J., Gruber, A. J., Kinnersley, B., Chubb, D., Frangou, A., Caravagna, G., Noyvert, B., Lakatos, E., Wood, H. M., Thorn, S., Culliford, R., Arnedo-Pac, C., Househam, J., Cross, W., Sud, A., Law, P., Leathlobhair, M. N., Hawari, A., Woolley, C., ... Houlston, R. S. (2024). The genomic landscape of 2,023 colorectal cancers. *Nature, 633*(8028), 127–136. https://doi.org/10.1038/s41586-024-07747-9

7. Eren, Z., Ozkurt, H., Unyıldız, M., Kazak, M., Gunay, E., Cifci, T., Basarili, K., & Tugcu, H. (2012). Colorectal cancer following negative colonoscopy: Is 5-year screening the correct interval to recommend? *Surgical Endoscopy, 27*(2), 542–547. https://doi.org/10.1007/s00464-012-2543-6

8. Froicu, E.-M., Oniciuc, O.-M., Afrăsânie, V.-A., Marinca, M.-V., Riondino, S., Dumitrescu, E. A., Alexa-Stratulat, T., Radu, I., Miron, L., Bacoanu, G., Poroch, V., & Gafton, B. (2024). The use of artificial intelligence in predicting

chemotherapy-induced toxicities in metastatic colorectal cancer: A data-driven approach for personalized oncology. *Diagnostics, 14*(18), Article 2074. https://doi.org/10.3390/diagnostics14182074

9. Ganesh, K., Stadler, Z. K., Cercek, A., Mendelsohn, R. B., Shia, J., Segal, N. H., & Diaz, L. A., Jr. (2019). Immunotherapy in colorectal cancer: Rationale, challenges and potential. *Nature Reviews Gastroenterology & Hepatology, 16*(6), 361–375. https://doi.org/10.1038/s41575-019-0126-x

10. Hassan, C., Spadaccini, M., Iannone, A., Maselli, R., Jovani, M., Chandrasekar, V. T., Antonelli, G., Yu, H., Areia, M., Dinis-Ribeiro, M., Bhandari, P., Sharma, P., Rex, D. K., Rösch, T., Wallace, M., & Repici, A. (2021). Performance of artificial intelligence in colonoscopy for adenoma and polyp detection: A systematic review and meta-analysis. *Gastrointestinal Endoscopy, 93*(1), 77–85.e6. https://doi.org/10.1016/j.gie.2020.06.059

11. Heald, B., Hampel, H., Church, J., Dudley, B., Hall, M. J., Mork, M. E., Singh, A., Stoffel, E., Stoll, J., You, Y. N., Yurgelun, M. B., Kupfer, S. S., & Collaborative Group of the Americas on Inherited Gastrointestinal Cancer. (2020). Collaborative Group of the Americas on Inherited Gastrointestinal Cancer position statement on multigene panel testing for patients with colorectal cancer and/or polyposis. *Familial Cancer, 19*(3), 223–239. https://doi.org/10.1007/s10689-020-00170-9

12. Hildebrand, L. A., Pierce, C. J., Dennis, M., Paracha, M., & Maoz, A. (2021). Artificial intelligence for histology-based detection of microsatellite instability and

prediction of response to immunotherapy in colorectal cancer. *Cancers, 13*(3), Article 391. https://doi.org/10.3390/cancers13030391

13. Imperiale, T. F., Ransohoff, D. F., Itzkowitz, S. H., Levin, T. R., Lavin, P., Lidgard, G. P., Ahlquist, D. A., & Berger, B. M. (2014). Multitarget stool DNA testing for colorectal-cancer screening. *New England Journal of Medicine, 370*(14), 1287–1297. https://doi.org/10.1056/NEJMoa1311194
14. Liao, J., Li, X., Gan, Y., Han, S., Rong, P., Wang, W., Li, W., & Zhou, L. (2023). Artificial intelligence assists precision medicine in cancer treatment. *Frontiers in Oncology, 12*, Article 998222. https://doi.org/10.3389/fonc.2022.998222
15. Ma, G. X., Shive, S. E., Wang, M. Q., & Tan, Y. (2009). Cancer screening behaviors and barriers in Asian Americans. *American Journal of Health Behavior, 33*(6), 650–660. https://doi.org/10.5993/ajhb.33.6.3
16. Mayo Clinic. (2024). *AI-assisted colonoscopies reduce miss rate by 50 percent.* https://www.mayoclinic.org/medical-professionals/cancer/news/ai-assisted-colonoscopies-reduce-miss-rate-by-50-percent/mac-20536196
17. Melkonian, S. C., Jim, M. A., Haverkamp, D., Wiggins, C. L., McCollum, J., White, M. C., Kaur, J. S., & Espey, D. K. (2019). Disparities in cancer incidence and trends among American Indians and Alaska Natives in the United States, 2010-2015. *Cancer Epidemiology, Biomarkers & Prevention, 28*(10), 1604–1611. https://doi.org/10.1158/1055-9965.EPI-19-0288

18. National Cancer Institute. (2023). *Genetic testing for inherited cancer susceptibility syndromes.* National Institutes of Health. https://www.cancer.gov/about-cancer/causes-prevention/genetics/genetic-testing-fact-sheet

19. Nunes, L., Li, F., Wu, M., Luo, T., Hammarström, K., Torell, E., Ljuslinder, I., Mezheyeuski, A., Edqvist, P. H., Glimelius, B., Palmqvist, R., Öfverholm, E., Smedby, K. E., & Sjöblom, T. (2024). Prognostic genome and transcriptome signatures in colorectal cancers. *Nature, 632*(8025), 600–607. https://doi.org/10.1038/s41586-024-07769-3

20. Repici, A., Badalamenti, M., Maselli, R., Correale, L., Radaelli, F., Rondonotti, E., Ferrara, E., Spadaccini, M., Alkandari, A., Fugazza, A., Anderloni, A., Galtieri, P. A., Pellegatta, G., Carrara, S., Di Leo, M., Craviotto, V., Lamonaca, L., Lorenzetti, R., Andrealli, A., Antonelli, G., ... Hassan, C. (2020). Efficacy of real-time computer-aided detection of colorectal neoplasia in a randomized trial. *Gastroenterology, 159*(2), 512–520.e7. https://doi.org/10.1053/j.gastro.2020.04.062

21. Russo, V., Lallo, E., Munnia, A., Spedicato, M., Messerini, L., D'Aurizio, R., Cerrani, E. G., Brunelli, G., Galvano, A., Russo, A., Landini, I., Morabito, F., Gattini, V., Peluso, M., & EuResist Network GEIE. (2022). Artificial intelligence predictive models of response to cytotoxic chemotherapy alone or combined to targeted therapy for metastatic colorectal cancer patients: A systematic review and meta-analysis. *Cancers, 14*(16), Article 4012. https://doi.org/10.3390/cancers14164012

22. Shaukat, A., Kahi, C. J., Burke, C. A., Rabeneck, L., Sauer, B. G., & Rex, D. K. (2021). ACG Clinical Guidelines: Colorectal cancer screening 2021. *American Journal of Gastroenterology, 116*(3), 458–479. https://doi.org/10.14309/ajg.0000000000001122

23. Siegel, R. L., Wagle, N. S., Cercek, A., Smith, R. A., & Jemal, A. (2023). Colorectal cancer statistics, 2023. *CA: A Cancer Journal for Clinicians, 73*(3), 233–254. https://doi.org/10.3322/caac.21772

24. Syngal, S., Brand, R. E., Church, J. M., Giardiello, F. M., Hampel, H. L., Burt, R. W., & American College of Gastroenterology. (2015). ACG clinical guideline: Genetic testing and management of hereditary gastrointestinal cancer syndromes. *American Journal of Gastroenterology, 110*(2), 223–262. https://doi.org/10.1038/ajg.2014.435

25. Theimer, S. (2023, February 28). *Mayo Clinic Healthcare expert: Artificial intelligence improves colonoscopy accuracy*. Mayo Clinic News Network. https://newsnetwork.mayoclinic.org/discussion/mayo-clinic-healthcare-expert-artificial-intelligence-improves-colonoscopy-accuracy/

26. Wallace, M. B., Sharma, P., Bhandari, P., East, J., Antonelli, G., Lorenzetti, R., Vieth, M., Speranza, I., Spadaccini, M., Desai, M., Lukens, F. J., Babameto, G., Batista, D., Singh, D., Palmer, W., Ramirez, F., Palmer, R., Lunsford, T., Ruff, K., Bird-Liebermann, E., ... Hassan, C. (2022). Impact of artificial intelligence on miss rate of colorectal neoplasia. *Gastroenterology, 163*(1), 295–304.e5. https://doi.org/10.1053/j.gastro.2022.03.007

27. Yale School of Medicine. (2024). *AI-assisted colonoscopy: New research and guidelines for clinical use.* https://medicine.yale.edu/news-article/ai-assisted-colonoscopy-research-guidelines/

28. Yin, Z., Yao, C., Zhang, L., & Qi, S. (2023). Application of artificial intelligence in diagnosis and treatment of colorectal cancer: A novel prospect. *Frontiers in Medicine, 10*, Article 1128084. https://doi.org/10.3389/fmed.2023.1128084

Lung Cancer and AI: Your Ally in Prevention and Early Detection

1. American Cancer Society. (2025a). *Key statistics for lung cancer*. https://www.cancer.org/cancer/lung-cancer/about/key-statistics.html

2. American Cancer Society. (2025b). *Lung cancer risk factors.* https://www.cancer.org/cancer/lung-cancer/causes-risks-prevention/risk-factors.html

3. American Lung Association. (2024). *State of lung cancer report.* https://www.lung.org/research/state-of-lung-cancer

4. Bendotti, H., Lawler, S., Chan, G. C., Gartner, C., Ireland, D., & Marshall, H. M. (2023). Conversational artificial intelligence interventions to support smoking cessation: A systematic review and meta-analysis. *Digital Health, 9*, Article 20552076231211634. https://doi.org/10.1177/20552076231211634

5. Birdsey, J., Cornelius, M., Jamal, A., Park-Lee, E., Cooper, M. R., Wang, J., Sawdey, M. D., Cullen, K. A., & Neff, L. (2023). Tobacco product use among U.S. middle

and high school students - National Youth Tobacco Survey, 2023. *Morbidity and Mortality Weekly Report, 72*(44), 1173–1182. https://doi.org/10.15585/mmwr.mm7244a1

6. Cahill, K., Lindson-Hawley, N., Thomas, K. H., Fanshawe, T. R., & Lancaster, T. (2016). Nicotine receptor partial agonists for smoking cessation. *Cochrane Database of Systematic Reviews, 5*, Article CD006103. https://doi.org/10.1002/14651858.CD006103.pub7
7. Callaghan, R. C., Allebeck, P., & Sidorchuk, A. (2013). Marijuana use and risk of lung cancer: A 40-year cohort study. *Cancer Causes & Control, 24*(10), 1811–1820. https://doi.org/10.1007/s10552-013-0259-0
8. Centers for Disease Control and Prevention. (2024a, June 7). *American Indian and Alaska Native people.* Tips from Former Smokers. https://www.cdc.gov/tobacco/campaign/tips/groups/american-indian-alaska-native.html
9. Centers for Disease Control and Prevention. (2024b). *Unfair and unjust practices and conditions harm African American people and drive health disparities.* https://www.cdc.gov/tobacco-health-equity/collection/african-american-unfair-and-unjust.html
10. Chung, S., Baumlin, N., Dennis, J. S., Moore, R., Salathe, S. F., Whitney, P. L., Sabater, J., Abraham, W. M., Kim, M. D., & Salathe, M. (2019). Electronic cigarette vapor with nicotine causes airway mucociliary dysfunction preferentially via TRPA1 receptors. *American Journal of Respiratory and Critical Care Medicine, 200*(9), 1134–1145. https://doi.org/10.1164/rccm.201811-2087OC

11. Environmental Protection Agency. (2023). *Health risk of radon*. https://www.epa.gov/radon/health-risk-radon

12. Gotts, J. E., Jordt, S. E., McConnell, R., & Tarran, R. (2019). What are the respiratory effects of e-cigarettes? *BMJ, 366*, Article l5275. https://doi.org/10.1136/bmj.l5275

13. Graham, A. L., Amato, M. S., Cha, S., Jacobs, M. A., Bottcher, M. M., & Papandonatos, G. D. (2021). Effectiveness of a vaping cessation text message program among young adult e-cigarette users: A randomized clinical trial. *JAMA Internal Medicine, 181*(7), 923–930. https://doi.org/10.1001/jamainternmed.2021.1793

14. Hartmann-Boyce, J., Chepkin, S. C., Ye, W., Bullen, C., & Lancaster, T. (2018). Nicotine replacement therapy versus control for smoking cessation. *Cochrane Database of Systematic Reviews, 2018*(5), Article CD000146. https://doi.org/10.1002/14651858.CD000146.pub5

15. Jonas, D. E., Reuland, D. S., Reddy, S. M., Nagle, M., Clark, S. D., Weber, R. P., Enyioha, C., Malo, T. L., Brenner, A. T., Armstrong, C., Coker-Schwimmer, M., Middleton, J. C., Voisin, C., & Harris, R. P. (2021). Screening for lung cancer with low-dose computed tomography: Updated evidence report and systematic review for the US Preventive Services Task Force. *JAMA, 325*(10), 971–987. https://doi.org/10.1001/jama.2021.0377

16. Kuperberg, S. J., & Christiani, D. C. (2025). Artificial intelligence-based methods: The path forward in achieving equity in lung cancer screening and evaluation. *Cancer Innovation, 4*(3), Article e70019. https://doi.org/10.1002/cai2.70019

17. Li, Y., Xiao, X., Han, Y., Gorlova, O., Qian, D., Leighl, N., Johansen, J. S., Barnett, M., Chen, C., Goodman, G., Cox, A., Taylor, F., Woll, P., Wichmann, H. E., Manz, J., Muley, T., Risch, A., Rosenberger, A., Arnold, S. M., ... Amos, C. I. (2018). Genome-wide interaction study of smoking behavior and non-small cell lung cancer risk in Caucasian population. *Carcinogenesis, 39*(3), 336–346. https://doi.org/10.1093/carcin/bgx113

18. Lin, Y., Zhang, W., Chen, L., Wu, X., & Li, J. (2025). The feasibility and cost-effectiveness of implementing mobile low-dose computed tomography with an AI-based diagnostic system in underserved populations. *BMC Cancer, 25*, Article 279. https://doi.org/10.1186/s12885-025-13710-2

19. Lindson, N., Chepkin, S. C., Ye, W., Fanshawe, T. R., Bullen, C., & Hartmann-Boyce, J. (2019). Different doses, durations and modes of delivery of nicotine replacement therapy for smoking cessation. *Cochrane Database of Systematic Reviews, 4*, Article CD013308. https://doi.org/10.1002/14651858.CD013308

20. Nam, J. G., Park, S., Hwang, E. J., Lee, J. H., Jin, K. N., Lim, K. Y., Vu, T. H., Sohn, J. H., Hwang, S., Goo, J. M., & Park, C. M. (2019). Development and validation of deep learning-based automatic detection algorithm for malignant pulmonary nodules on chest radiographs. *Radiology, 290*(1), 218–228. https://doi.org/10.1148/radiol.2018180237

21. National Health Service. (2023, March 27). *Lung cancer screening*. https://www.nhs.uk/tests-and-treatments/lung-cancer-screening/

22. Olano-Espinosa, E., Avila-Tomas, J. F., Minue-Lorenzo, C., Matilla-Pardo, B., Serrano, M. E. S., Martinez-Suberviola, F. J., Monedero-Valles, B., Mendive-Arbeloa, J. M., Barragan-Casas, J. M., Sanchez-Gomez, L. M., Rodriguez-Rodriguez, E., Rodriguez-Arias, F., Lopez-Rodriguez, J. A., Gil-Conesa, M., Martin-Ferrer, R., Gonzalez-Quintana, P., Martinez-Martinez, R., Sabater-Hernandez, D., Motero-Martin, A., & Minue-Garcia, B. (2022). Effectiveness of a conversational chatbot (Dejal@bot) for the adult population to quit smoking: Pragmatic, multicenter, controlled, randomized clinical trial in primary care. *JMIR mHealth and uHealth, 10*(6), Article e34273. https://doi.org/10.2196/34273

23. Pandit, A., & Radkani, S. (2022). The impact of artificial intelligence on health equity in oncology: Scoping review. *Journal of Medical Internet Research, 24*(11), Article e39748. https://doi.org/10.2196/39748

24. Public Health England. (2007, November 1). *Radon: indicative atlas in England and Wales.* https://www.gov.uk/government/publications/radon-indicative-atlas-in-england-and-wales

25. Sim, Y., Chung, M. J., Kotter, E., Yune, S., Kim, M., Do, S., Han, K., Kim, H., Yang, S., Lee, D. J., & Choi, B. W. (2020). Deep convolutional neural network-based software improves radiologist detection of malignant lung nodules on chest radiographs. *Radiology, 294*(1), 199–209. https://doi.org/10.1148/radiol.2019182465

26. Stead, L. F., Koilpillai, P., Fanshawe, T. R., & Lancaster, T. (2016). Combined pharmacotherapy and behavioural

interventions for smoking cessation. *Cochrane Database of Systematic Reviews, 3*, Article CD008286. https://doi.org/10.1002/14651858.CD008286.pub3

27. Truth Initiative. (2020, May 28). *Tobacco use in the Asian American community*. https://truthinitiative.org/research-resources/targeted-communities/tobacco-use-asian-american-community

28. U.S. Preventive Services Task Force. (2021). Interventions for tobacco smoking cessation in adults: US Preventive Services Task Force recommendation statement. *JAMA, 325*(3), 265–279. https://doi.org/10.1001/jama.2020.25019

29. Webb Hooper, M., Carpenter, K. M., Salmon, E. E., & Resnicow, K. (2023). Enhancing tobacco quitline outcomes for African American adults: An RCT of a culturally specific intervention. *American Journal of Preventive Medicine, 65*(6), 964–972. https://doi.org/10.1016/j.amepre.2023.06.005

30. Whittaker, R., Dobson, R., & Garner, K. (2022). Chatbots for smoking cessation: Scoping review. *Journal of Medical Internet Research, 24*(9), Article e35556. https://doi.org/10.2196/35556

## Breathing Room: AI's Boost for Your Lungs

1. Alpha-1 Foundation. (2024). *Alpha-1 antitrypsin deficiency*. https://www.alpha1.org

2. American Lung Association. (n.d.). *How your lungs get the job done*. https://www.lung.org/blog/how-your-lungs-work

3. Centers for Disease Control and Prevention. (2021). *Asthma FastStats.* https://www.cdc.gov/asthma/data/asthma-faststats.html

4. Centers for Disease Control and Prevention. (2023). Trends in the prevalence of chronic obstructive pulmonary disease—United States, 2011–2021. *Morbidity and Mortality Weekly Report, 72*(46), 1250–1256. https://doi.org/10.15585/mmwr.mm7246a1

5. Gaudet, M., Cheminant, M. A., & Plourde, G. (2022). Recent advances in vitamin D implications in chronic respiratory diseases. *Respiratory Research, 23*(1), Article 252. https://doi.org/10.1186/s12931-022-02147-x

6. National Geographic. (2021, May 4). *Lungs information and facts.* https://www.nationalgeographic.com/science/article/lungs

7. Topalovic, M., Das, N., Burgel, P. R., Daenen, M., Derom, E., Haenebalcke, C., Janssen, R., Kerstjens, H. A. M., Liistro, G., Louis, R., Ninane, V., Pison, C., Schlesser, M., Vercauter, P., Vogelmeier, C. F., Wouters, E., Wynants, J., & Troosters, T. (2019). Artificial intelligence outperforms pulmonologists in the interpretation of pulmonary function tests. *European Respiratory Journal, 53*(4), Article 1801660. https://doi.org/10.1183/13993003.01660-2018

8. Yang, P., Sun, Z., Krowka, M. J., Aubry, M. C., Bamlet, W. R., Wampfler, J. A., Thibodeau, S. N., Katzmann, J. A., Allen, M. S., Midthun, D. E., Marks, R. S., & de Andrade, M. (2008). Alpha1-antitrypsin deficiency carriers, tobacco smoke, chronic obstructive pulmonary

disease, and lung cancer risk. *JAMA Internal Medicine, 168*(10), 1097–1103. https://doi.org/10.1001/archinte.168.10.1097

## Infectious Diseases and AI: Staying Ahead of Hidden Threats

1. BioFire Diagnostics. (2025, March 16–22). *BioFire syndromic trends: South region gastrointestinal report.* https://clinical.syndromictrends.com
2. bioMérieux. (2023). *BIOFIRE® respiratory 2.1 (RP2.1) panel & respiratory 2.1 plus (RP2.1plus) panel.* https://www.biomerieux.com/corp/en/our-offer/clinical-products/biofire-respiratory-2-1-panels.html
3. Centers for Disease Control and Prevention. (2024a). *Hepatitis C information.* https://www.cdc.gov/hepatitis/hcv/index.htm
4. Centers for Disease Control and Prevention. (2024b). *Lyme disease data and surveillance.* https://www.cdc.gov/lyme/data-research/facts-stats/index.html
5. Centers for Disease Control and Prevention. (2024c). *Shingles (herpes zoster) vaccination.* https://www.cdc.gov/shingles/vaccines/index.html
6. Centers for Disease Control and Prevention. (2024d). *Tuberculosis (TB) statistics. https://www.cdc.gov/tb/statistics/index.html*Cen
7. Centers for Disease Control and Prevention. (2023). *Viral hepatitis surveillance report—United States, 2021.* https://www.cdc.gov/hepatitis-surveillance-2021/about/?CDC_AAref_Val=https://www.cdc.gov/hepatitis/statistics/2021surveillance/index.htm

8. Hofmeister, M. G., Rosenthal, E. M., Barker, L. K., Rosenberg, E. S., Barranco, M. A., Hall, E. W., Edlin, B. R., Mermin, J., Ward, J. W., & Ryerson, A. B. (2019). Estimating prevalence of hepatitis C virus infection in the United States, 2013–2016. *Hepatology*, *69*(3), 1020–1031. https://doi.org/10.1002/hep.30297

9. Kilgore, P. E., Kruszon-Moran, D., Seward, J. F., Jumaan, A., Van Loon, F. P., Forghani, B., McQuillan, G. M., Wharton, M., Fehrs, L. J., Cossen, C. K., & Hadler, S. C. (2003). Varicella in Americans from NHANES III: Implications for control through routine immunization. *Journal of Medical Virology*, *70*(Suppl 1), S111–S118. https://doi.org/10.1002/jmv.10364

10. Kugeler, K. J., Schwartz, A. M., Delorey, M. J., Mead, P. S., & Hinckley, A. F. (2021). Estimating the frequency of Lyme disease diagnoses, United States, 2010–2018. *Emerging Infectious Diseases*, *27*(2), 616–619. https://doi.org/10.3201/eid2702.202731

11. MD Anderson Cancer Center. (2020). *Hepatitis C and liver cancer: What you need to know*. https://www.mdanderson.org/publications/focused-on-health/HepatitisC-liver-cancer-What-you-need-to-know.h16Z1591413.html

12. Schmid, D. S., & Jumaan, A. O. (2010). Impact of varicella vaccine on varicella-zoster virus dynamics. *Clinical Microbiology Reviews*, *23*(1), 202–217. https://doi.org/10.1128/CMR.00031-09

## Part 3: Personalized Prevention: AI Tools for Proactive Health Management

### Your AI Medication Assistant: Another Layer of Protection

1. Barnsteiner, J. H. (2008). Medication reconciliation. In R. G. Hughes (Ed.), *Patient safety and quality: An evidence-based handbook for nurses*. Agency for Healthcare Research and Quality. https://www.ncbi.nlm.nih.gov/books/NBK2648/

2. Bonaudo, M., Martorana, M., Dimonte, V., D'Alfonso, A., Fornero, G., Politano, G., & Gianino, M. M. (2018). Medication discrepancies across multiple care transitions: A retrospective longitudinal cohort study in Italy. *PLOS ONE, 13*(1), Article e0191028. https://doi.org/10.1371/journal.pone.0191028

3. Heyworth, L., Clark, J., Marcello, T. B., Paquin, A. M., Stewart, M., Archambeault, C., & Simon, S. R. (2013). Aligning medication reconciliation and secure messaging: qualitative study of primary care providers' perspectives. *Journal of Medical Internet Research, 15*(12), Article e264. https://doi.org/10.2196/jmir.2793

4. Ong, J. C. L., Lim, Z. W., Chew, H. S. J., Tan, K. B., & Car, J. (2025). A scoping review on generative AI and large language models in mitigating medication-related harm. *NPJ Digital Medicine, 8*, Article 3. https://doi.org/10.1038/s41746-025-01565-7

## Supplements and AI: A Smart Path to Better Health

1. Aroda, V. R., Edelstein, S. L., Goldberg, R. B., Knowler, W. C., Marcovina, S. M., Orchard, T. J., Bray, G. A., Schade, D. S., Temprosa, M. G., White, N. H., & Crandall, J. P. (2016). Long-term metformin use and vitamin B12 deficiency in the Diabetes Prevention Program Outcomes Study. *The Journal of Clinical Endocrinology & Metabolism, 101*(4), 1754–1761. https://doi.org/10.1210/jc.2015-3754

2. Asher, G. N., Corbett, A. H., & Hawke, R. L. (2017). Common herbal-drug interactions: What the primary care provider needs to know. *American Family Physician, 96*(2), 101–107. https://www.aafp.org/pubs/afp/issues/2017/0715/p101.html

3. Ferraro, P. M., Curhan, G. C., Gambaro, G., & Taylor, E. N. (2016). Total, dietary, and supplemental vitamin C intake and risk of incident kidney stones. *American Journal of Kidney Diseases, 67*(3), 400–407. https://doi.org/10.1053/j.ajkd.2015.09.005

4. Frye, R. E., Sequeira, J. M., Quadros, E. V., James, S. J., & Rossignol, D. A. (2013). Cerebral folate receptor autoantibodies in autism spectrum disorder. Molecular Psychiatry, 18(3), 369-381. https://doi.org/10.1038/mp.2011.175

5. Goodman, M., & Chen, X. H. (1996). Are U.S. lower normal B12 limits too low? *Journal of the American Geriatrics Society, 44*(10), 1274–1275. https://doi.org/10.1111/j.1532-5415.1996.tb01389.x

6. Grant, W. B., Wimalawansa, S. J., Płudowski, P., & Cheng, R. Z. (2025). Vitamin D: Evidence-based health benefits and recommendations for population guidelines. *Nutrients, 17*(2), Article 277. https://doi.org/10.3390/nu17020277

7. Hicks, J. K., Sangkuhl, K., Swen, J. J., Ellingrod, V. L., Müller, D. J., Shimoda, K., Bishop, J. R., Kharasch, E. D., Skaar, T. C., Gaedigk, A., Dunnenberger, H. M., Klein, T. E., Caudle, K. E., & Stingl, J. C. (2017). Clinical Pharmacogenetics Implementation Consortium guideline (CPIC) for CYP2D6 and CYP2C19 genotypes and dosing of tricyclic antidepressants: 2016 update. *Clinical Pharmacology & Therapeutics, 102*(1), 37–44. https://doi.org/10.1002/cpt.597

8. Holick, M. F. (2007). Vitamin D deficiency. *New England Journal of Medicine, 357*(3), 266–281. https://doi.org/10.1056/NEJMra070553

9. Holick, M. F., Binkley, N. C., Bischoff-Ferrari, H. A., Gordon, C. M., Hanley, D. A., Heaney, R. P., Murad, M. H., & Weaver, C. M. (2011). Evaluation, treatment, and prevention of vitamin D deficiency: An Endocrine Society clinical practice guideline. *Journal of Clinical Endocrinology & Metabolism, 96*(7), 1911–1930. https://doi.org/10.1210/jc.2011-0385

10. Institute of Medicine. (1998). *Dietary reference intakes for thiamin, riboflavin, niacin, vitamin B6, folate, vitamin B12, pantothenic acid, biotin, and choline.* National Academies Press. https://doi.org/10.17226/6015

11. Mason, M., Cho, Y., Rayo, J., Gong, Y., Harris, M., & Jiang, Y. (2022). Technologies for medication adherence monitoring and technology assessment criteria: Narrative review. *JMIR mHealth and uHealth, 10*(3), Article e35157. https://doi.org/10.2196/35157

12. Mitsuyama, Y., & Kogoh, H. (1988). Serum and cerebrospinal fluid vitamin B12 levels in demented patients with CH3-B12 treatment—preliminary study. *Japanese Journal of Psychiatry and Neurology, 42*(1), 65–71. https://doi.org/10.1111/j.1440-1819.1988.tb01957.x

13. Mozaffarian, D., & Wu, J. H. (2011). Omega-3 fatty acids and cardiovascular disease: Effects on risk factors, molecular pathways, and clinical events. Journal of the *American College of Cardiology, 58*(20), 2047–2067. https://doi.org/10.1016/j.jacc.2011.06.063

14. Ordovas, J. M., Ferguson, L. R., Tai, E. S., & Mathers, J. C. (2018). Personalized nutrition and health. BMJ, 361, k2173. https://doi.org/10.1136/bmj.k2173

15. Oulhaj, A., Jernerén, F., Refsum, H., Smith, A. D., & de Jager, C. A. (2016). Omega-3 fatty acid status enhances the prevention of cognitive decline by B vitamins in mild cognitive impairment. *Journal of Alzheimer's Disease, 50*(2), 547–557. https://doi.org/10.3233/JAD-150777

16. Pacholok, S. M., & Stuart, J. J. (2011). *Could it be B12? An epidemic of misdiagnoses* (2nd ed.). Quill Driver Books.

17. Rajman, I., Chwalek, K., & Sinclair, D. A. (2018). Therapeutic potential of NAD-boosting molecules: The in vivo evidence. *Cell Metabolism, 27*(3), 529–547. https://doi.org/10.1016/j.cmet.2018.02.011

18. Rossignol, D. A., & Frye, R. E. (2021). Cerebral folate deficiency, folate receptor alpha autoantibodies and leucovorin (folinic acid) treatment in autism spectrum disorders: A systematic review and meta-analysis. Journal of Personalized Medicine, 11(11), 1141. https://doi.org/10.3390/jpm11111141

19. Zhang, Y., Li, X., Zou, D., Liu, W., Yang, J., Zhu, N., Huo, L., Wang, M., Hong, J., Wu, P., Ren, G., & Ning, G. (2008). Treatment of type 2 diabetes and dyslipidemia with the natural plant alkaloid berberine. *The Journal of Clinical Endocrinology & Metabolism, 93*(7), 2559–2565. https://doi.org/10.1210/jc.2007-2404

### Preventive Medicine and Longevity

1. Adan, A. (2012). Cognitive performance and dehydration. *Journal of the American College of Nutrition, 31*(2), 71–78. https://doi.org/10.1080/07315724.2012.10720011

2. Barzilai, N., Crandall, J. P., Kritchevsky, S. B., & Espeland, M. A. (2016). Metformin as a tool to target aging. *Cell Metabolism, 23*(6), 1060–1065. https://doi.org/10.1016/j.cmet.2016.05.011

3. Cain, T., Brinsley, J., Bennett, H., Nelson, M., Maher, C., & Singh, B. (2025). Effects of cold-water immersion on health and wellbeing: A systematic review and meta-analysis. *PLOS One, 20*(1), Article e0317615. https://doi.org/10.1371/journal.pone.0317615

4. Campisi, J., Kapahi, P., Lithgow, G. J., Melov, S., Newman, J. C., & Verdin, E. (2019). From discoveries in ageing research to therapeutics for healthy ageing.

*Nature, 571*(7764), 183–192. https://doi.org/10.1038/s41586-019-1365-2

5. Espeland, D., de Weerd, L., & Mercer, J. B. (2022). Health effects of voluntary exposure to cold water – a continuing subject of debate. *International Journal of Circumpolar Health, 81*(1), Article 2111789. https://doi.org/10.1080/22423982.2022.2111789
6. Fries, J. F. (1980). Aging, natural death, and the compression of morbidity. *New England Journal of Medicine, 303*(3), 130–135. https://doi.org/10.1056/NEJM198007173030304
7. Fries, J. F., Bruce, B., & Chakravarty, E. (2011). Compression of morbidity 1980-2011: A focused review of paradigms and progress. *Journal of Aging Research, 2011*, Article 261702. https://pmc.ncbi.nlm.nih.gov/articles/PMC3163136/
8. Gamel, S.A., Talaat, F.M. (2024). SleepSmart: an IoT-enabled continual learning algorithm for intelligent sleep enhancement. *Neural Computing and Applications, 36*, 4293–4309. https://doi.org/10.1007/s00521-023-09310-5
9. Golden, R. N., Gaynes, B. N., Ekstrom, R. D., Hamer, R. M., Jacobsen, F. M., Suppes, T., Wisner, K. L., & Nemeroff, C. B. (2005). The efficacy of light therapy in the treatment of mood disorders: A review and meta-analysis of the evidence. *American Journal of Psychiatry, 162*(4), 656–662. https://doi.org/10.1176/appi.ajp.162.4.656
10. Huberman, A. (2022, April 4). Using light (sunlight, blue light & red light) to optimize health [Audio podcast episode]. In *Huberman Lab*. Scicomm Media. https://

www.hubermanlab.com/episode/using-light-sunlight-blue-light-and-red-light-to-optimize-health

11. Imai, S., & Guarente, L. (2014). NAD+ and sirtuins in aging and disease. *Trends in Cell Biology, 24*(8), 464–471. https://doi.org/10.1016/j.tcb.2014.04.002
12. Kapoor, A., Narayanan, S., & Manchanda, P. (2025). *Does access to human coaches lead to more weight loss than with AI coaches alone?* (Working Paper No. 4070). Stanford Graduate School of Business. https://www.gsb.stanford.edu/faculty-research/working-papers/does-access-human-coaches-lead-more-weight-loss-ai-coaches-alone
13. Laukkanen, T., Kunutsor, S. K., Kauhanen, J., & Laukkanen, J. A. (2018). Sauna bathing is associated with reduced cardiovascular mortality and improves risk prediction in men and women: A prospective cohort study. *BMC Medicine, 16*(1), Article 219. https://doi.org/10.1186/s12916-018-1198-0
14. Lee, L. L., Mulvaney, C. A., Wong, Y. K. Y., Chan, E. S., Watson, M. C., & Lin, H. H. (2021). Walking for hypertension. *Cochrane Database of Systematic Reviews, 2021*(2), Article CD008823. https://doi.org/10.1002/14651858.CD008823.pub2
15. Lovato, N., & Lack, L. (2010). The effects of napping on cognitive functioning. *Progress in Brain Research, 185*, 155–166. https://doi.org/10.1016/B978-0-444-53702-7.00009-9
16. Ma, X., Yue, Z. Q., Gong, Z. Q., Zhang, H., Duan, N. Y., Shi, Y. T., Wei, G. X., & Li, Y. F. (2017). The effect of diaphragmatic breathing on attention, negative

affect and stress in healthy adults. *Frontiers in Psychology*, *8*, Article 874. https://doi.org/10.3389/fpsyg.2017.00874

17. Magnuson, C. D., & Barnett, L. A. (2013). The playful advantage: How playfulness enhances coping with stress. *Leisure Sciences*, *35*(2), 129–144. https://doi.org/10.1080/01490400.2013.761905

18. Murphy, M. H., Blair, S. N., & Murtagh, E. M. (2009). Accumulated versus continuous exercise for health benefit: A review of empirical studies. *Sports Medicine*, *39*(1), 29–43. https://doi.org/10.2165/00007256-200939010-00003

19. Proyer, R. T. (2013). The well-being of playful adults: Adult playfulness, subjective well-being, physical well-being, and the pursuit of enjoyable activities. *European Journal of Humour Research*, *1*(1), 84–98. https://doi.org/10.7592/EJHR2013.1.1.proyer

20. Rosekind, M. R., Smith, R. M., Miller, D. L., Co, E. L., Gregory, , KB, Webbon, L. L., Gander, P. H., & Lebacqz, J. V. (1995). Alertness management: strategic naps in operational settings. *Journal of Sleep Research*, *4*(S2), 62–66. https://doi.org/10.1111/j.1365-2869.1995.tb00229.x

21. Sinclair, D. A., & LaPlante, M. D. (2019). *Lifespan: Why we age—and why we don't have to.* Atria Books.

22. Steger, F. L., Donnelly, J. E., Hull, H. R., Li, X., Hu, J., & Sullivan, D. K. (2022). Retention, fasting patterns, and weight loss with an intermittent fasting app: Large-scale, 52-week observational study. *JMIR mHealth*

*and uHealth, 10*(10), Article e35896. https://doi.org/10.2196/35896

23. Walker, M. (2017). *Why we sleep: Unlocking the power of sleep and dreams*. Scribner.

24. Wilson, K. (2025). *Hack your body, heal your mind* [Audiobook]. BBC Studios. https://www.audible.com/pd/Hack-your-Body-Heal-your-Mind-Audiobook/B0DNKLBZKZ

25. Wittbrodt, M. T., & Millard-Stafford, M. (2018). Dehydration impairs cognitive performance: A meta-analysis. *Medicine and Science in Sports and Exercise, 50*(11), 2360–2368. https://doi.org/10.1249/MSS.0000000000001682

26. Yi, L., Maier, A. B., Tao, R., Lin, Z., Vaidya, A., Pendse, S., Thasma, S., Andhalkar, S., Avhad, G., & Kumbhare, D. (2023). The efficacy and safety of β-nicotinamide mononucleotide (NMN) supplementation in healthy middle-aged adults: A randomized, multicenter, double-blind, placebo-controlled, parallel-group, dose-dependent clinical trial. *GeroScience, 45*(1), 29–43. https://doi.org/10.1007/s11357-022-00705-1

27. Zeevi, D., Korem, T., Zmora, N., Israeli, D., Rothschild, D., Weinberger, A., Ben-Yacov, O., Lador, D., Avnit-Sagi, T., Lotan-Pompan, M., Suez, J., Mahdi, J. A., Matot, E., Malka, G., Kosower, N., Rein, M., Zilberman-Schapira, G., Dohnalová, L., Pevsner-Fischer, M., ... Segal, E. (2015). Personalized nutrition by prediction of glycemic responses. *Cell, 163*(5), 1079–1094. https://doi.org/10.1016/j.cell.2015.11.001

## AI as Your Helper

1. Esteva, A., Kuprel, B., Novoa, R. A., Ko, J., Swetter, S. M., Blau, H. M., & Thrun, S. (2017). Dermatologist-level classification of skin cancer with deep neural networks. *Nature*, *542*(7639), 115–118. https://doi.org/10.1038/nature21056

2. Makary, M. (2024). *Blind spots: When medicine gets it wrong, and what it means for our health.* Bloomsbury Publishing.

3. National Comprehensive Cancer Network. (2024). *NCCN Clinical Practice Guidelines in Oncology: Breast cancer* (Version 4.2024). https://www.nccn.org/guidelines/guidelines-detail?category=1&id=1419

4. Peck, M., Moffat, D., Latham, B., & Badrick, T. (2018). Review of diagnostic error in anatomical pathology and the role and value of second opinions in error prevention. *Journal of Clinical Pathology*, *71*(11), 995–1000. https://doi.org/10.1136/jclinpath-2018-205226

5. Rajpurkar, P., Chen, E., Banerjee, O., & Topol, E. J. (2022). AI in health and medicine. *Nature Medicine*, *28*(1), 31–38. https://doi.org/10.1038/s41591-021-01614-0

6. Topol, E. J. (2019). *Deep medicine: How artificial intelligence can make healthcare human again.* Basic Books.

7. Tyson, M. (2025, October 29). Grieving family uses AI chatbot to cut hospital bill from $195,000 to $33,000—family says Claude highlighted duplicative charges, improper coding, and other violations. Tom's Hardware. https://www.tomshardware.com/tech-industry/artificial-intelligence/

grieving-family-uses-ai-chatbot-to-cut-hospital-bill-from-usd195-000-to-usd33-000-family-says-claude-highlighted-duplicative-charges-improper-coding-and-other-violations

## Conclusion

1. American Diabetes Association. (2024). Standards of Care in Diabetes—2024. *Diabetes Care, 47*(Suppl 1). https://doi.org/10.2337/dc24-SINT

2. An, J. E., Kim, K. H., Park, S. J., Seo, S. E., Kim, J., Ha, S., Bae, J., & Kwon, O. S. (2022). Wearable cortisol Aptasensor for simple and rapid real-time monitoring. *ACS sensors, 7*(1), 99–108. https://doi.org/10.1021/acssensors.1c01734

3. Apple Inc. (2024). *Using Apple Watch for arrhythmia detection.* Apple Support. https://support.apple.com/guide/watch/apda3c3c7f5e/watchos

4. Attia, Z. I., Kapa, S., Lopez-Jimenez, F., McKie, P. M., Ladewig, D. J., Satam, G., Pellikka, P. A., Enriquez-Sarano, M., Noseworthy, P. A., Munger, T. M., Asirvatham, S. J., Scott, C. G., Carter, R. E., & Friedman, P. A. (2019). Screening for cardiac contractile dysfunction using an artificial intelligence–enabled electrocardiogram. *Nature Medicine, 25*(1), 70–74. https://doi.org/10.1038/s41591-018-0240-2

5. Attia, Z. I., Noseworthy, P. A., Lopez-Jimenez, F., Asirvatham, S. J., Deshmukh, A. J., Gersh, B. J., Carter, R. E., Yao, X., Rabinstein, A. A., Erickson, B. J., Kapa, S., & Friedman, P. A. (2019). An artificial intelligence-enabled ECG algorithm for the identification of patients

with atrial fibrillation during sinus rhythm: A retrospective analysis of outcome prediction. *The Lancet, 394*(10201), 861–867. https://doi.org/10.1016/S0140-6736(19)31721-0

6. Bekiari, E., Kitsios, K., Thabit, H., Tauschmann, M., Athanasiadou, E., Karagiannis, T., Haidich, A.-B., Hovorka, R., & Tsapas, A. (2018). Artificial pancreas treatment for outpatients with type 1 diabetes: Systematic review and meta-analysis. *BMJ, 361,* Article k1310. https://doi.org/10.1136/bmj.k1310
7. Buysse, D. J. (2014). Sleep health: Can we define it? Does it matter? *Sleep, 37*(1), 9–17. https://doi.org/10.5665/sleep.3298
8. Chaudhary, U., Birbaumer, N., & Ramos-Murguialday, A. (2016). Brain-computer interfaces in the completely locked-in state and chronic stroke. *Progress in Brain Research, 228*, 131–161. https://doi.org/10.1016/bs.pbr.2016.04.019
9. Huang, S. M., Wu, F. H., Ma, K. J., et al. (2025). Individual and integrated indexes of inflammation predicting the risks of mental disorders - statistical analysis and artificial neural network. *BMC Psychiatry, 25*, Article 226. https://doi.org/10.1186/s12888-025-06652-3
10. Kiss, H., Örlős, Z., Gellért, Á., Megyesfalvi, Z., Mikáczó, A., Sárközi, A., Vaskó, A., Miklós, Z., & Horváth, I. (2023). Exhaled biomarkers for point-of-care diagnosis: Recent advances and new challenges in breathomics. *Micromachines, 14*(2), Article 391. https://doi.org/10.3390/mi14020391

11. Lee, I. M., Shiroma, E. J., Evenson, K. R., Kamada, M., LaCroix, A. Z., & Buring, J. E. (2018). Accelerometer-measured physical activity and sedentary behavior in relation to all-cause mortality: The Women's Health Study. *Circulation, 137*(2), 203–205. https://doi.org/10.1161/CIRCULATIONAHA.117.031300

12. Makary, M. (2024). Blind spots: *When medicine gets it wrong, and what it means for our health.* Bloomsbury Publishing.

13. Nazarian, S., Lam, K., Darzi, A., & Ashrafian, H. (2021). Diagnostic accuracy of smartwatches for the detection of cardiac arrhythmia: Systematic review and meta-analysis. *Journal of Medical Internet Research, 23*(8), Article e28974. https://doi.org/10.2196/28974

14. Obermeyer, Z., Powers, B., Vogeli, C., & Mullainathan, S. (2019). Dissecting racial bias in an algorithm used to manage the health of populations. *Science, 366*(6464), 447–453. https://doi.org/10.1126/science.aax2342

15. Quer, G., Arnaout, R., Henne, M., & Arnaout, R. (2021). Machine learning and the future of cardiovascular care: JACC state-of-the-art review. *Journal of the American College of Cardiology, 77*(3), 300–313. https://doi.org/10.1016/j.jacc.2020.11.030

16. Rajpurkar, P., Chen, E., Banerjee, O., & Topol, E. J. (2022). AI in health and medicine. *Nature Medicine, 28*(1), 31–38. https://doi.org/10.1038/s41591-021-01614-0

17. Ridker, P. M., Moorthy, M. V., Cook, N. R., Rifai, N., Lee, I. M., & Buring, J. E. (2024). Inflammation, cholesterol, lipoprotein(a), and 30-year cardiovascular

outcomes in women. *New England Journal of Medicine. 391*(22), 2087–2097. https://doi.org/10.1056/NEJMoa2405182

18. Ruedy, K. J., Parkin, C. G., Riddlesworth, T. D., Graham, C., & DIAMOND Study Group. (2017). Continuous glucose monitoring in older adults with type 1 and type 2 diabetes using multiple daily injections of insulin: Results from the DIAMOND trial. *Journal of Diabetes Science and Technology, 11*(6), 1138–1146. https://doi.org/10.1177/1932296817704445
19. Topol, E. J. (2019). *Deep medicine: How artificial intelligence can make healthcare human again.* Basic Books.
20. Vamathevan, J., Clark, D., Czodrowski, P., Dunham, I., Ferran, E., Lee, G., Li, B., Madabhushi, A., Shah, P., Spitzer, M., & Zhao, S. (2019). Applications of machine learning in drug discovery and development. *Nature Reviews Drug Discovery, 18*, 463–477. https://doi.org/10.1038/s41573-019-0024-5
21. Wang, F., & Wang, J. D. (2021). Investing preventive care and economic development in ageing societies: Empirical evidences from OECD countries. *Health Economics Review, 11*, Article 18. https://doi.org/10.1186/s13561-021-00321-3
22. Wang, M., Yang, Y., Min, J., Song, Y., Tu, J., Mukasa, D., Ye, C., Xu, C., Heflin, N., McCune, J. S., Hsiai, T. K., Li, Z., & Gao, W. (2022). A wearable electrochemical biosensor for the monitoring of metabolites and nutrients. *Nature Biomedical Engineering*, 6(11), 1225–1235. https://doi.org/10.1038/s41551-022-00916-z

23. Willett, F. R., Avansino, D. T., Hochberg, L. R., Henderson, J. M., & Shenoy, K. V. (2021). High-performance brain-to-text communication via handwriting. *Nature, 593*(7858), 249–254. https://doi.org/10.1038/s41586-021-03506-2

24. World Economic Forum. (2018, May 15). *Four ways AI can slash healthcare costs around the world.* https://www.weforum.org/stories/2018/05/four-ways-ai-is-bringing-down-the-cost-of-healthcare/

25. Yin, L., Moon, J. M., Sempionatto, J. R., Lin, M., Cao, X., Bo, J., Lou, X., Xie, B., Sun, A., Liu, Y., Lee, C., De la Paz, E., Kurniawan, J. F., Xu, Y., Chen, G., He, X., Xu, M., Salvalaglio, M., Paul, R., ... Wang, J. (2022). A stretchable epidermal sweat sensing platform with integrated flexible electrochemical sensors and electrochromic display. *Nature Electronics, 5*(10), 694–705. https://doi.org/10.1038/s41928-022-00843-6

26. Zhao, Y., Wang, B., Hojaiji, H., Wang, Z., Lin, S., Yeung, C., Lin, H., Nguyen, P., Chiu, K., Salahi, K., Cheng, X., Tan, J., Cerrillos, B., & Emaminejad, S. (2022). A wearable freestanding cortisol-sensing system. *Science Advances, 8*(1), Article eabk0967. https://doi.org/10.1126/sciadv.abk0967

# INTERNS

## DOMINIC GIOVANETTI

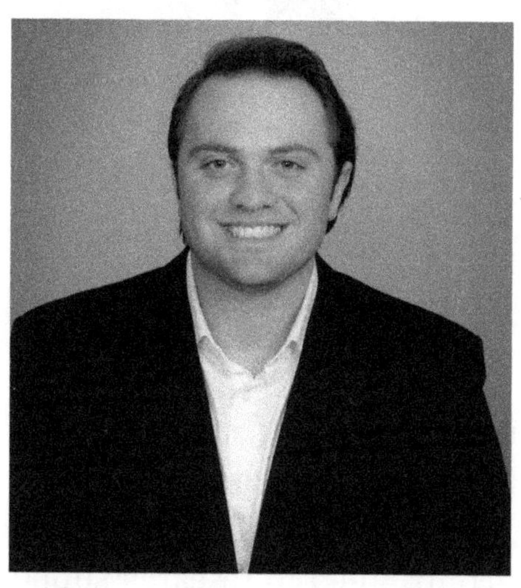

Dominic Giovanetti is a first-year medical student at the Lake Erie College of Osteopathic Medicine at Seton Hill University and is certified by the National Board of Public Health Examiners. He holds a degree in chemistry with a focus in biochemistry and biotechnology from the University of South Florida, where he also earned his Master of Public Health from the university's highly regarded program.

During his studies, Dominic worked with Dr. Earl Campazzi, Jr. to help complete this publication and conducted liver health research in collaboration with the University of South Florida while working at Encompass Health. In his free time, he enjoys exercising, spending time with family, watching sports, and cooking.

# NIKA WOLFS

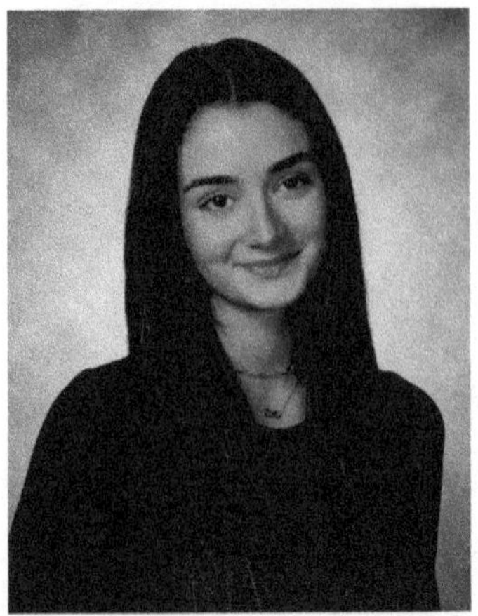

Nika Wolfs is entering her senior year at Cornell University, majoring in human development, with plans to apply to medical school to begin in Fall 2027. During her summer internship, she contributed to research supporting this book and gained valuable experience observing in the office.

# LIA LOVE

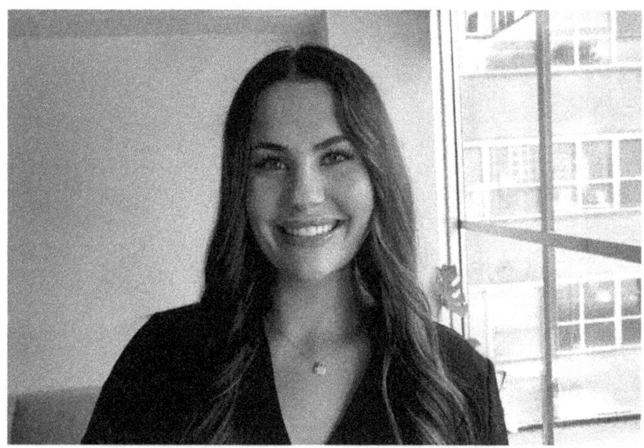

Lia Love is a neuroscience graduate from the University of Michigan and current researcher in the neurosurgery department at the University of Pennsylvania. She investigates how traumatic brain injury contributes to long-term cognitive dysfunction, such as post-traumatic epilepsy. She is pursuing a career in medicine with the goal of becoming a physician whose practice is rooted in empathy, advocacy, and improving patients' quality of life.

During the COVID-19 pandemic, Lia joined Dr. Campazzi's practice as a medical assistant while contributing to this book's research. While assisting with patient care, she dove into research articles and tackled the books Dr. Campazzi assigned.

## REAGAN DALY

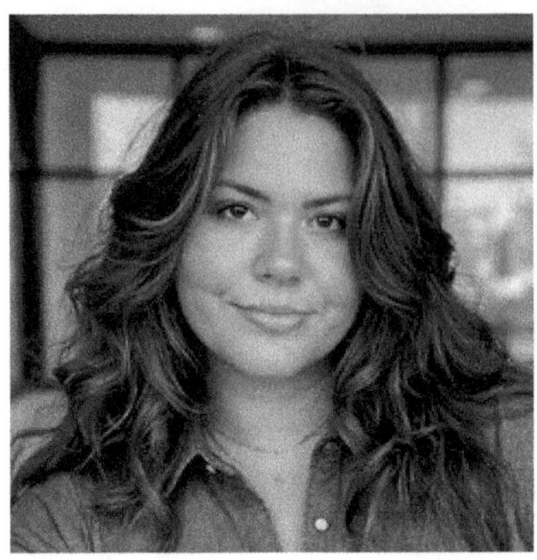

Reagan Daly was a premedical student in Thessaloniki, Greece, before finishing college at Boston University. She lives in St. Thomas in the U.S. Virgin Islands.

While at The Lawrenceville School, Reagan worked as an intern for Dr. Campazzi. She helped gather research about preventing disease and dementia for this book and learned about AI in healthcare.

During her internship, Reagan watched the doctors, nurses, and other health workers at Dr. Campazzi's practice. She saw how patients benefited when doctors focus on keeping people healthy instead of just treating them when they get sick.

Reagan wants to use what she learns to improve healthcare in the U.S. Virgin Islands through better public health programs.